Finding Joy in Alzheimer's: New Hope for Caregivers

Marie Marley, PhD

Daniel C. Potts, MD, FAAN

Finding Joy in Alzheimer's: New Hope for Caregivers
By Marie Marley, PhD, and Daniel C. Potts, MD, FAAN

© 2015 by Marie Marley, PhD, and Daniel C. Potts, MD, FAAN

Editors: Carol Bradley Bursack, BA; Ellen W. Potts, MBA; and Mary Theobald, MBA

Cover Art: Painting by Lester E. Potts, Jr., Daniel C. Potts' father. This painting was created after Daniel's father was diagnosed with Alzheimer's.

All rights reserved. No part of this book may be used or reproduced in any manner whatsoever without written permission, except for brief quotations embodied in critical articles and reviews.

First Edition
ISBN: 9781512321975

Joseph Peterson Books
Kansas City

Marie

To Ed
and to
Marjorie Rentz and Clarissa Rentz
for their love and support

To those dedicated caregivers who give so much of
themselves every day

To all those special people living with Alzheimer's
and other dementias

Daniel

To the memory of my father, Lester

To the honor of my mother, Ethelda

To all who give of themselves to enrich the lives
of people with dementia

To those courageous souls living with a diagnosis of Alzheimer's
or another dementia

Foreword

"Alzheimer's" and "hope" aren't usually words people put into the same sentence. It's a disease which at this moment – November 2015 – has no cure. But there is a lot of hope. Marie Marley and Daniel Potts have managed to find light in the midst of the darkness that can prevail while caring for a loved one with Alzheimer's.

Unlike most books on the topic, which focus on the difficulties of caring for those with the illness, *Finding Joy in Alzheimer's: New Hope for Caregivers* shines a light on the uplifting and inspiring moments you can experience and share while caring for someone and navigating this mind-blowing disease.

This groundbreaking volume, written by two former caregivers, will show those still dealing with this disease day in and day out how to come to terms with their loved one's condition so that they can free their mind and heart to embrace and enjoy the time they spend together. As a child of Alzheimer's – my father, Sargent Shriver died of the disease in 2011 – I know first-hand how important it is to find moments of grace and joy even while the person you love is losing control of his or her own mind.

Marie and Daniel smartly divided this book into three parts, which will show you how people living with Alzheimer's can still enjoy life, give insight into overcoming the devil called "denial," letting go of resentment and the role grief plays on our journey to acceptance. As everyone associated with Alzheimer's must eventually accept, in order to move forward with the person your loved one has become, you must acknowledge and grieve the person they used to be. Grief is something I still experience over the loss of my father. He had the brightest mind I've ever encountered, but while we were living with his disease, I learned how to enjoy the new person he was becoming and was able to have interactions I'll treasure for the rest of my life.

Between tips on how to interact and visit with people with dementia and stories from their personal experiences, the guidance and real-life tools offered in these pages will provide immeasurable support for the oh-so-important caretakers who themselves are offering everyday support on what I call "the front lines of humanity."

I have hope that we will one day find a cure and wipe out Alzheimer's. But, until then, it is books like this, offering hope, guidance and community that will help us all to navigate the ever-shifting tides that accompany an Alzheimer's diagnosis – for the patients, families and caretakers. Hats off to Marie and Daniel for tackling this much-needed topic.

    Maria Shriver

CONTENTS

Dedications 5
Foreword by Maria Shriver 7
Table of Contents 9
Introduction 13
A Word About Terminology Used in This Book 15

PART I: The First Step: Make Peace With Alzheimer's

Chapter 1: People With Alzheimer's Can Still Enjoy Life 18
Chapter 2: Is Alzheimer's Always Depressing? The Authors Think Not 23
Chapter 3: Alzheimer's and the Devil Called 'Denial' 26
Chapter 4: Overcoming Denial 33
Chapter 5: Five Especially Difficult Situations to Accept 38
Chapter 6: The Role of Grief on the Journey to Acceptance 52
Chapter 7: Making Peace With God 55

Part II: Tips for Interacting With People Who Have Alzheimer's

Chapter 8: Tips for Interacting 60
Chapter 9: How to Behave When Visiting in a Facility 74

PART III: Stories About Our Personal Joyous Relationships and Visits

Chapter 10: Meet Ed and Meet Marie's 'Ladies'..........................80

Chapter 11: Meet Daniel's Dad...99

Chapter 12: Stories About Love and Acceptance 122
- The 'Lee-tle' Yellow One
- I Love You
- Expecting a Gift
- Two Men With Alzheimer's Connect
- The Innate Human Capacity to Feel Joy
- I Like That Kind
- A Special Relationship
- The Art of Listening
- The Poetic Voice of Alzheimer's
- Love Remembered Despite Alzheimer's

Chapter 13: Humorous Stories 157
- Laughing With Lola
- A Brief Walk on the Light Side of Dementia
- Bring Me Vodka!
- Enough!

- People Who Have Alzheimer's Can Say the Darndest Things
- The Spelling Bee
- Maria's New Walker
- To the Mortuary!

Chapter 14: Stories About Special Activities..................184
- Please Wear a Tux
- I'm Proud of Your Art!
- 'Conducting' a Visit
- The Little Stuffed Animals
- Art With Mary
- The Beep Game
- Visiting Miss Daisy
- A Puppy in a Pocket
- Gifts Can Bring Joy to a Person Who Has Alzheimer's
- Skipping Rocks
- The Alzheimer's Perspective on the Birds and the Bees
- Puppy's Magical Visit to a Memory Care Facility

Chapter 15: Stories About Moments of Lucidity.................226
- Introduction
- An Intuitive Knowing

- You'll Get the Job
- Dogs Are Very Selective
- Moments of Clarity
- Wearing it for Death
- You're Always in My Heart

Acknowledgments..248
About the Authors...250
Appendix: Works Cited..253

Introduction

Marie (co-author of this book) volunteers to visit some ladies with Alzheimer's at a memory care facility near her home. One day Marie was visiting Ruth when Ruth asked if Marie would like a cookie.

Marie patted her ample tummy and asked, "Do I look like I need a cookie?"

Ruth then said, "Oh, you're just settling!"

This is just one of many joyous moments Marie experienced in her relationship with Ruth.

In Part I of this book, the authors support their premise that people with Alzheimer's can still enjoy life (Chapter 1). Then they look at the issue of whether Alzheimer's is always depressing (Chapter 2). After that, there are chapters about denial and the importance of overcoming it (Chapters 3 and 4). Next, the authors discuss five especially difficult situations to accept (Chapter 5). Then, they talk about the role of grief on the journey to acceptance (Chapter 6). This is followed by a discussion about making peace with God in the midst of the reality of Alzheimer's (Chapter 7).

In Part II, 55 tips for visiting loved ones who have Alzheimer's are presented (Chapter 8), and then there are tips for how to behave when visiting a person in a facility (Chapter 9).

Part III introduces the people with whom Marie and Daniel (the co-authors of this book) had joyous relationships and visits (Chapters 10 and 11), and Chapters 12 to 15 contain stories about joyful visits they had with these people.

It has been said in the literature on Alzheimer's that "If you have seen one person with Alzheimer's, you have seen one person with Alzheimer's," meaning that each person with the disease is unique. However, there tend to be some commonalities, and those are what the authors discuss throughout this book.

A Word About Terminology Used in This Book

The authors focus on having joyous relationships and visits with people living with Alzheimer's. 'Relationship' refers to interactions with individuals who have the disease, but more importantly, it is used to describe the mutual love, affection, and acceptance one can have with them. Life, in all its fullness, can only be experienced when we have relationships.

Another term used frequently is 'visit.' 'Visit' refers to visiting someone in an assisted living setting or in a memory care facility, nursing home, or hospice facility. 'Visit' also applies to interactions between staff in a daycare center and those who have Alzheimer's, as well as to caregivers interacting with their loved ones at home.

'Facility' is used for any type of facility where people with Alzheimer's may live: assisted living, memory care, nursing home, hospice care, and others.

'Care partner' and 'caregiver' are used throughout the book to refer to family caregivers or other unpaid caregivers, as opposed to professional ones in facilities. 'Loved one' indicates a person with Alzheimer's.

Though the authors have chosen to focus on their experiences in relationships with people who have Alzheimer's, their stories and advice can be generalized to include individuals who have other causes of dementia. 'Dementia' is a term that refers to one's loss of cognitive abilities to the degree that it interferes with daily life. Alzheimer's is the most common cause of dementia, though there are many other possible causes. The terms 'Alzheimer's' or

'Alzheimer's disease' are used in this book to refer to Alzheimer's and other types of dementia.

Finally, 'he,' 'him' and 'his' are used to refer to both genders.

PART I

The First Step: Make Peace With Alzheimer's

Chapter 1: People With Alzheimer's Can Still Enjoy Life

<u>Thankfulness</u>

I saw a marquis today that read, "Thankfulness begins with a good memory." I disagree. Those without a good memory can still be thankful. All it takes to be thankful is to be alive and present each moment to the wonder and utter enjoyment of this gift of life that we have all been given, and an ever-awakening awareness of the divine flame that dances in all things, at all times, and calls us to join in the dance.

Daniel

Many people regard Alzheimer's as a cruel and devastating disease that destroys its 'victims.' One that robs them of their very humanity. There's virtually nothing more chilling than to realize a loved one has developed this difficult illness and to ponder all the diagnosis means.

Care partners may fall into a period of deep depression and despondence when the diagnosis is made. Anticipatory grief also may develop. One realizes that life as it had been planned has been lost forever. Companionship and intimacy may appear to have vanished.

The caregiver can also become angry at the situation and angry at God for the painful reality that his loved one has developed Alzheimer's. The caregiver may sometimes even be angry at his loved one who has the disorder. It isn't unusual for care partners to pass through a period when they don't even want to visit their loved ones anymore.

Yes, it seems that Alzheimer's is a devastating illness and that those who have it can never again enjoy life. When Marie interviewed and read the books of several experts on the disease, however, a somewhat different picture emerged. The experts unanimously agreed that although Alzheimer's is a terrible disease, people who have it can and do retain the capacity to enjoy life.

According to Virginia Bell and David Troxel, writing in *The Best Friends Approach to Alzheimer's Care*, "Too much attention has been paid to the 'tragic side' of Alzheimer's disease. This is a terrible disease. Yet, by dwelling on the negative it is too easy to victimize people with the illness and settle for lower standards of care."

Teepa Snow, a nationally renowned expert on Alzheimer's caregiving, also believes that people with Alzheimer's can enjoy life. In an interview, she told Marie, "Yes. Almost all people with dementia, even those in the later stages of the disease, can enjoy life if they have the right support and environment."

The entire book, *Creating Moments of Joy: A Journal for Caregivers*, by Jolene Brackey, is dedicated to this issue. Brackey states, "I have a vision. A vision that we will soon look beyond the challenges of Alzheimer's disease and focus more of our energy on creating moments of joy." She adds, "We are not able to create a perfectly wonderful day with [people who have Alzheimer's], but it is absolutely attainable to create perfectly wonderful moments—moments that put smiles on their faces, a twinkle in their eyes, or trigger [pleasant] memories."

Carole Larkin, owner of Third Age Services in the Dallas/Ft. Worth area, is a geriatric care manager who specializes in helping families with dementia issues. When Marie asked Larkin whether she thinks individuals living with Alzheimer's can still enjoy life, she answered, "Absolutely. They can and do enjoy life. That enjoyment, when it happens, is moment by moment—pretty much the same way we enjoy life."

Tom and Karen Brenner, a husband and wife team of Alzheimer's caregiving experts, train family members, professional caregivers, and medical staff in the use of cutting-edge interventions for persons who have dementia. Tom answered the same question by saying, "Yes. And their enjoyment in life is based, in part, on our enjoyment of them. It's like a swinging door: it goes both ways."

Karen added, "We believe we can reach all people with Alzheimer's, including those whom others consider unable to communicate in any way at all. It's almost always possible to communicate, even with people who have lost their verbal skills."

People in Various Stages of the Disease

People in the Early Stage of Alzheimer's

In the early stages of the disease, activities enjoyed before Alzheimer's can be an opportunity for shared interaction. However, some activities may need to be adjusted to accommodate the loved one's diminishing mental capacity. For example, consider a simple card game instead of bridge, checkers instead of chess. Another example of a simplified activity is jigsaw puzzles with fewer and larger pieces. (Such puzzles are available from puzzlestoremember.org.)

People with Mid-Stage Alzheimer's

In the middle stage, those who have Alzheimer's have lost more of their mental and some of their social skills. While it's fine to do the old standbys, such as looking at old pictures or watching movies together, those are somewhat passive activities. With a little thought, more active ways to spend time together can be found. This might include handing the person 'props' that can be played with together. The key words here are 'play' and 'together.'

People in the Latest Stage of the Disease

Snow, in partnership with Senior Helpers, an in-home care company, developed 'Senior Gems,' a system that classifies people with Alzheimer's into six categories, each named after a gem. The categories are Sapphires, Diamonds, Emeralds, Ambers, Rubies, and Pearls. The 'Gems' table shows the basic characteristics of individuals at each stage of the disorder and provides tips for interacting with them. Pearls are at the latest stage of the disease.

According to the 'Gems' table, Pearls:

> "Like pleasant sounds and familiar voices. They also like to feel warm and comfortable. For people in this category it's beneficial to read or talk to them about good memories. They might not understand your words, but your voice will be soothing. You

might also bring a new extra soft blanket or sweater for them to wrap up in or brush their hair and apply lotion to their skin."

Yes, people with Alzheimer's can, and indeed do, still have the capacity to enjoy life.

Chapter 2: Is Alzheimer's Always Depressing? The Authors Think Not

<u>Hope</u>

Each interaction we have with another person, no matter how brief or casual, presents an opportunity to share the hope that is within us.

Daniel

Alzheimer's is a deadly serious illness. But does 'serious' mean that it is always horrible and depressing? It *can* be horrible and depressing. It can be tragic and painful. It can be heartbreaking and terrible. Even agonizing and excruciating.

But is it always that way? The authors think not. They believe that to some extent, it depends on the attitude of the beholder. The following vignette illustrates this point.

John is distraught when he visits his wife, Jean. First of all, he finds the facility depressing. While walking to his wife's room, he passes several residents sitting in wheelchairs. Most are either staring into space or their heads are hanging down and they appear to be dozing. "What a waste of human life," he thinks.

Worse still is his wife's condition. She can't bathe or dress herself. She needs help eating. She carries a baby doll around with her everywhere she goes. She acts as though it's a real baby. John has tried and tried to convince her it's just a doll, and he's tried to get her to give it up. All to no avail.

Jill is another regular visitor to the same facility. When she walks down the hall and sees the residents staring into space, she says 'hello' to them in the tone of voice you'd use when greeting a friend. In many cases, they lift their heads, look surprised, smile, and return her greeting. They're surprised because usually no one talks to them that way!

Jill's mother, the past president of a major university, can often be found playing Bingo, which she can't play unless one of the aides helps her. Her mother's other favorite activity is the sing-along sessions held every Tuesday and Thursday.

Jill's reaction to the situation, however, is very different than John's. Sometimes Jill arrives during the Bingo game and sits beside her mother as her mother is playing. Instead of thinking about how much her mother's mental capacity has declined, she notes that her mother has a smile on her face. Jill is so happy there are still things her mother enjoys.

Although her mother usually doesn't recognize Jill, it's obvious that her mother enjoys Jill's visits. As far as the incontinence garments her mother wears, Jill isn't upset by them. There's nothing inherently distressing about these garments. Infants wear them, and that isn't depressing to anyone.

To a great extent, one's attitude about a person with Alzheimer's influences how one views that person. If a care partner is in denial and tries to insist that his loved one talk and behave like a person without the condition, he will be miserable every time he visits.

If people dwell on what their loved ones can't do rather than what they still can do, visiting will be painful. If they focus on comparing their loved one's current mental state to his previous one, they will suffer, and this may cause the loved one to suffer as well.

If caregivers think of their own unhappiness about a given issue rather than their loved ones' reaction to the same issue, they will never be able to accept the illness. They will never be at peace with the situation.

Sometimes, the best thing to do when feeling upset about something is to ask whether the person living with Alzheimer's is upset by it. An individual may be distressed, for example, because the aides don't style his mother's hair very well. Instead, he should ask himself if his mother is upset by it. If not, then he should let it go.

Jill enjoys her visits because she accepts her mother just as she is. She doesn't try to change her. She has a relationship with her at her current level—not her previous level.

No, Alzheimer's doesn't always have to be depressing.

Chapter 3: Alzheimer's and the Devil Called 'Denial'

<u>Love them as they are</u>

To care for someone with dementia, one has to let go of his mental construct of who that person was to embrace the reality of who the person is now. The essential core of someone with Alzheimer's remains the same, and that is where one should strive for connection. This will always require some degree of selfless compassion and empathy, which will result in personal growth through the power of love.

Daniel

Alzheimer's is, above all, an insidious disease. Its distressing symptoms often begin so mildly and progress so slowly that it's easy for friends and family members to deny the symptoms until sometimes there's a 'defining incident,' an incident so upsetting and bizarre that not even a spouse, child, or other caregiver can ignore it or explain it away. Various disconcerting 'defining incidents' have been reported in the literature. Some people get lost driving home and end up bewildered and many miles away. Some leave the house in their pajamas, and some fail to recognize a close friend or family member. These are just a few of hundreds of examples.

Yet the disease typically starts with symptoms of little or no significance. Not being able to come up with a common word. Mixing up someone's name. Forgetting to turn off the stove. Things we all do from time to time. However, for the person just beginning the Alzheimer's journey, these problems begin to occur more and more often, which confuses and worries both the person with the symptoms and the care partner.

Years may pass between the earliest occasional disquieting confusion and the 'defining incident.' During those years, the person with Alzheimer's may annoy or even anger friends and family members by being late, forgetting important appointments, being short-tempered, being unable to perform routine tasks, and exhibiting a whole variety of other troublesome behaviors.

As people developing the disease slowly decline, they typically struggle to adjust and continue functioning. This takes extreme mental effort, often leading to anger and agitation. During this time, those developing Alzheimer's are also usually in denial, realizing something is wrong and trying to understand it in any way possible that doesn't involve the words 'Alzheimer's' or 'dementia.'

Marie's Experience With Denial

It was obvious to Marie that Ed, her beloved Romanian soul mate of 30 years, was worried about possibly having Alzheimer's. He used humor as a coping mechanism. He ended every medical visit by pronouncing loudly, "At least it isn't Alzheimer's!" Then he laughed heartily.

Marie's denial of Ed's symptoms was particularly strong. She worked hard to come up with explanations for each symptom. When Ed repeatedly confused the name of his bank with the name of the grocery store, she thought it was just a normal sign of aging. When he couldn't pay his bills properly, she thought he'd just had too much to drink that evening.

When he completely forgot a phone conversation they'd just had, she honestly couldn't come up with a logical excuse, so she just pushed the incident to the back of her mind and soon forgot about it. There were many events she ignored over a period of years.

When Ed's symptoms became more severe, Marie still made excuses for him. The time he got lost driving to the corner gas station, she thought he was just temporarily confused. Even when he was found driving on the wrong side of the road one night, she decided it only happened because he was driving at night—something his doctor said he shouldn't do because of his failing eyesight.

But a 'defining incident' finally occurred. One night Ed didn't know what a kitchen was and said that furthermore, he didn't have one. Considering this and all the other signs of Alzheimer's he'd been exhibiting, Marie finally had to face the cold, hard truth: Ed was most likely developing Alzheimer's. And her heart broke in that moment.

Daniel's Experience With Denial

Daniel's experience of denial with his father, Lester, was similar in many ways. The early changes were subtle. Daniel helped his mother, Lester's primary caregiver, care for Lester. She told Daniel about minor behavioral changes Lester exhibited. Both Daniel and his mother chalked up the changes to Lester getting older, going through life transitions, etc.

Then came delirium after a minor surgery, trouble keeping up with finances, and short-term memory loss. The 'defining incident' for Daniel came when his dad lost his job parking cars at a local office building. Unbeknownst to Daniel and his mother, Lester was losing cars, locking keys in cars, and getting lost in the parking deck, which upset his co-workers. They complained to his supervisor, and this resulted in Lester having to relinquish his job.

When Lester's supervisor met with Daniel about this, Daniel was taken by surprise, and a great sadness hit like a ton of bricks. In reality, even though Daniel is a neurologist experienced with treating people who have Alzheimer's, he had been in denial. Looking back, he says that the day his dad's supervisor visited was one of the hardest days of his life.

With the clarity of hindsight, and having spoken with many caregivers on the subject, the authors have concluded that the denial individuals experience when confronted with their loved ones' Alzheimer's has a lot to do with their own egos' desire to hold on to the image of the loved one they have in their mind.

Author Madeleine L'Engle said, "Because you're not what I would have you be, I blind myself to who, in truth, you are."

There is reality and then there is the perception of that reality. It is normal to create a mental impression of those with whom one has relationships, and that impression is in part dependent on past experiences with them, the needs the relationship has fulfilled, future expectations, etc. But when people are confronted with the Alzheimer's diagnosis, everything changes, including the very nature of their relationship with the person who has Alzheimer's.

In many ways, it is a kind of death, and when people confront death they do not usually accept it with serenity.

So denial can function as a defense against loss—the loss of the loved one as one knew him, the loss of the previous relationship with that person, and the loss of the part of one's self that is defined by the relationship.

The challenge is to learn to accept reality and not let that acceptance change the affection one has for the person living with Alzheimer's or one's own desire to maintain the relationship. It's important not to blind one's self to the true person beneath the disease. This individual remains, and no disease process can take that away. Because of this, relationships are always possible, no matter how advanced the loved one's condition.

People who notice consistent signs of confusion and forgetfulness in a loved one should not wait for a 'defining incident.' One early action to take is to review the Alzheimer's Association's 10 Signs of Dementia and ask whether their loved one has one or more of them:

1. Memory loss that disrupts daily life
2. Challenges in planning or solving problems
3. Difficulty completing familiar tasks at home, at work, and at leisure
4. Confusion with time or place
5. Difficulty understanding visual images and spatial relationships
6. New problems with words in speaking or writing
7. Losing things and the inability to retrace steps
8. Decreased or poor judgment

9. Withdrawal from work or social activities
10. Changes in mood and personality

The Alzheimer's Association web site (Alz.org) has additional information about each of these symptoms and explains how they differ from things 'normal people' do from time to time. Mostly, signs of Alzheimer's are a matter of how often the symptoms occur and how prominent they are.

It's easy to ignore these signs or fail to connect the dots, but when a person is showing the signs it's essential to dig deep into one's soul and find the emotional strength to get a medical evaluation as soon as possible. Doctors may determine that the cause of the memory problems is treatable, even curable.

If it is determined that a loved one is developing Alzheimer's, early detection gives the caregiver and the person with the illness time to prepare for the future and allows for appropriate medications to be prescribed, which often work better if started early. In addition, it allows the loved one to participate in long-range planning for his future, including financial planning, arranging legal affairs, and thinking about an eventual move to a care facility.

An early diagnosis also helps the caregiver and his friends and family members adjust to the loved one's condition, rather than becoming angry at that person's unusual actions and personality changes, which are often negative. Early diagnosis allows everyone to be more understanding and compassionate with the person developing the condition.

No one wants to be evaluated or have a loved one evaluated for Alzheimer's disease, but sometimes it has to be done—and the sooner the better.

Chapter 4: Overcoming Denial

<u>Caregiving</u>

Caregiving can bring out our best or worst qualities. What matter are connection, love for ourselves and another, acceptance, and forgiveness.

Daniel

Denial May Deprive Caregivers of Joy

One of Ed's former colleagues to whom he was exceedingly close—I'll call him George—was visiting Ed from out of town. One evening the two had a long talk about a wide range of topics, most of which involved George's professional concerns. The next day, Ed had no memory of the visit, let alone what they had discussed.

I had been telling George for months that Ed had Alzheimer's, but George never believed me. He thought Ed's memory problems were just due to normal aging. In short, he was in a state of deep denial.

George simply couldn't believe that Ed didn't remember their time together the previous evening. He tried to jog Ed's memory, but it didn't work. At all.

George was distressed. In fact, he spent all the rest of his time with Ed trying to refresh his memory of their talk. When it didn't work, he left for the airport to go home, upset and distraught.

What George didn't realize was that Ed would never remember their visit. It would have made more sense for them to spend their remaining time together discussing something else or experiencing their relationship in some other way. They could have had a pleasant—maybe even joyous—visit.

For example, they could have spent the time playing with the little stuffed animals Ed loved so much. Marie made this suggestion to George, and he dismissed it out of hand. He wasn't going to play with Ed and his stuffed animals. He felt it was beneath both his and Ed's dignity.

Unfortunately, George's refusal—or perhaps inability—to accept the fact that Ed's cognitive state was seriously impaired prevented them from moving on to something more pleasant.

As long as George was in this state of denial, he'd never know the joy Marie had with Ed and the little animals. He'd never see Ed smile and hear him laugh as Marie so often did when they played with them. He'd never know how much fun it was.

Marie's friend, Sandy, experienced a similar situation. Sandy's grandmother had dementia, and Sandy's mother was in denial. She kept trying to make her mother act 'normal.'

Sandy's grandmother kept asking, "Where are the girls?" Her tone of voice made it obvious that she was upset about not knowing where 'the girls' were. (Nobody quite knew what she meant by 'the girls.')

Sandy's mother kept trying (in vain) to explain that there were no girls. When this explanation didn't stop the question about the girls, Sandy's mother became upset. She tried and tried and tried, but nothing ever made her mother stop asking the question.

When Sandy came to visit, her grandmother asked her the same question: "Where are the girls?" Sandy didn't know what girls her grandmother was asking about, but she simply said, "They're in school, Grandma."

And that was the end of it, at least for a while. Sandy's grandmother stopped asking about the girls, and they went on to have a pleasant visit.

Whenever the issue of the girls arose, Sandy tried to explain to her mother that she should tell a similar white lie and get on with the visit —a visit in which they could experience a satisfying relationship.

Unfortunately, Sandy's mother, who was in deep denial, could never accept this advice, and she subsequently became depressed. She didn't really enjoy her relationship or her visits with her mother.

All too often caregivers are in denial. Hence, they spend their time trying to get a person with dementia to 'act normal.' Trying to get him to remember and do things he will never be able to remember or do.

This only leads to anger and frustration for the visitor and often for the person with Alzheimer's, as well.

It is much better to look for ways to have a relationship and interact at the level of a loved one rather than try to drag that person into one's world. Because the person with Alzheimer's can't function in the 'normal' world. One can only reach him and enjoy him in his world. At his level. In 'Alzheimer's world,' as Bob DeMarco, founder of the Alzheimer's Reading Room, calls it.

Those in denial about their loved ones' disease rarely know they're in denial. They believe that people with Alzheimer's can be 'normal' and remember things if they just try hard enough to make those people remember. Hence, it's difficult for caregivers to change the way they approach their relationships and how they spend time with their loved ones.

Denial is a serious problem; the solution is quite difficult. If a person interacts with someone who doesn't have Alzheimer's but who's forgotten something important, the natural thing is to try to jog their memory. Chances are they will remember. This is 'normal.'

If one tries the same thing with a person who has Alzheimer's, however, he will inevitably be disappointed. His efforts will fail. He will miss out on the joy he might have if he accepts the person's memory loss and finds some other way to connect. To connect on a level that could be meaningful to both him and his loved one.

Those who feel they may be in denial should try interacting in a way that focuses on the present moment rather than one that involves the memory of the person with Alzheimer's. They may be pleasantly surprised.

The First Steps: Make Peace With Alzheimer's and Learn to Love Again

It's one thing to finally overcome denial and realize a loved one has Alzheimer's. It's a completely different thing to accept that fact. After what can be months or even years of being in denial, most people finally realize Alzheimer's has struck.

Many people are never able to accept the situation. Some caregivers never come to terms with it. Some never become at peace with the diagnosis and all it means. They know in their brains that their loved one will never get better, but as hard as they try they can't accept this truth it in their hearts.

It's not uncommon to get caught in a trap. The bold truth is so painful that one may push it to the back of his mind. The situation may be so hurtful that one responds by refusing to think about it. The caregiver may stick his head in the sand and pretend nothing serious is wrong.

To come to terms with Alzheimer's one must first let go of the expectation that they'll find the previous person, and instead embrace the new person—just as he is in the present. Since that person will continue changing as time goes by, one must constantly let go of the old person and accept the new one.

Each day brings the opportunity to experience new life with a loved one who has Alzheimer's. It's necessary to fall in love again with the person as he is in the present and let go of the person one used to love. That person is never coming back. This is what it means to accept and make peace with Alzheimer's: to learn to let go and learn to love again. This will give the caregiver and the loved one a great gift.

Chapter 5: Five Especially Difficult Situations to Accept

<u>Acceptance</u>

Today, I will do my best to choose to accept life as it is, not as I would have it; to be thankful for opportunities, freedoms, people, and experiences that come my way; to forgive myself and others for past failures; to laugh some and take myself lightly; to relinquish control over situations I really don't control anyway; to keep a song in my ear, and try to leave everyone I meet a little better than I found them; to pray or meditate, be honest, stay humble, and remain grateful for the life and love that I have been given, realizing I have done nothing to deserve any of it. I will fail at all of the above, but I promise to keep trying today.

Daniel

Those who care for people with Alzheimer's must deal with several painful symptoms. These include memory loss, confusion, changes in personality (which can be negative), loss of interest in activities previously enjoyed, a general inability for self-care, eventual incontinence, and so many more.

Some of these are more difficult to accept than others. In this chapter, the authors discuss the five situations that are probably the most difficult of all with which to come to terms:

1. If the loved one has to be moved to a care facility
2. If the loved one no longer recognizes the caregiver
3. If the loved one finds a new love
4. If the loved one loses the ability to talk
5. If the loved one needs hospice care

Let's look at each of these in some detail.

1. If the Loved One Has to Be Moved to a Care Facility

The decision to place a loved one in a care facility can be a controversial and agonizing one. Many people dedicate themselves to taking care of their loved ones at home regardless of how difficult it is. Caregivers are on duty 24/7 and often become physically and emotionally exhausted. Research has shown that the health and cognitive function of people caring for those with Alzheimer's typically suffer.

Many persons say they would rather die than place their loved ones in an institution, but in some cases—not all—such placement actually may be the best solution for both caregivers and those with Alzheimer's.

Although people with Alzheimer's may have previously stated their adamant opposition to living in an assisted living, long-term care, or other facility, many with mid- to advanced-stage Alzheimer's will adjust—often sooner than their caregivers. They may even forget they moved.

The following issues should be considered before a placement decision is made.

- **The caregiver is not an expert at realizing when his loved one has a significant health problem that requires immediate medical attention.** This is probably the most important reason to place a loved one in a facility. Staff members in such facilities are trained to recognize physical health problems, and there are physicians on call who can immediately initiate treatment and/or refer the person with Alzheimer's to a specialist, if needed. In addition, staff members are likely to know whether the person needs to be sent to the emergency room and, if so, they can arrange for immediate transportation there.

- **The caregiver can't provide the amount of socialization a facility can.** People with Alzheimer's (and everyone for that matter) need to be around others for socialization. This typically improves their mood and sense of well-being. Residents of a facility have the opportunity to interact with staff and other residents on a daily—even hourly—basis. At home, they usually have fewer opportunities for socialization.

- **The caregiver can't provide the frequency and quality of activities a facility can.** Most memory care, long-term care, and specialty care assisted living facilities (SCALFs) have specially trained activity directors who devote 100% of their time to providing meaningful activities for residents, whereas the family caregiver might have difficulty providing activities. For example, group sing-alongs are therapeutic, but caregivers might not be able to organize these at home.

- **Caregivers are not experts at communicating and interacting with people living with Alzheimer's.** Those in the mid- to late-stages of Alzheimer's may exhibit challenging behaviors, largely because they can't express their feelings and needs by traditional means. Most personnel in facilities receive training for dealing with these behaviors and for learning how to identify and provide for unmet needs. Family caregivers may have problems handling these difficult situations, leading to stressful interactions for both the caregivers and their loved ones.

- **Placement may be the best solution for the caregiver and thus, ultimately, for his loved one as well.** This is another important reason to consider placing a loved one in a facility. Although the care partner may be staunchly dedicated to caring for his loved one at home, providing 24/7 care is exhausting. One simply can't provide the best care if one is burned out all the time. Staff in facilities are usually on duty for only eight hours at a time. They can have a good emotional rest before returning the next day, whereas a family caregiver will likely have very little, if any, respite. Another benefit of placement is that when people aren't on duty all day every day they can relax and enjoy their relationships with their loved ones.

The overall well-being of the person with dementia should be taken into account when deciding what to do. This will help assuage feelings of guilt and will probably improve the care that individual receives.

2. If the Loved One No Longer Recognizes the Caregiver

Most individuals who have a loved one with Alzheimer's dread the day when their loved one no longer recognizes them. Care partners may think that would be the most tragic situation possible. They consider it the disastrous end of their relationship.

When a loved one doesn't recognize his caregiver, the caregiver can experience unending, searing pain. Ultimately, however, the situation hurts the caregiver, but may not bother the person living with Alzheimer's. That should be what matters most.

The authors believe someone with Alzheimer's can still feel a bond with his caregiver even if he doesn't know precisely who that person is. But some caregivers are so upset when their loved ones don't recognize them, they don't see any reason to keep visiting. They figure it doesn't matter. However, there are several reasons why continuing to visit does matter:

- **The person may recognize the caregiver but may not be able to express it**

It's always possible that the person with Alzheimer's does recognize the caregiver but cannot show it in ways that are easy to recognize.

Marie had a personal experience that demonstrates this. Doris was one of the ladies Marie was assigned to visit at the memory care facility where she volunteers. Doris was so frail and her condition so advanced that the most Marie could do was hold Doris's hand and speak to her softly. Doris never responded.

Then one day as Marie was holding her hand, Doris put her other hand on Marie's arm and began caressing it. Marie had the distinct feeling that Doris remembered her.

- **The person may remember how often he is visited even if he no longer remembers his relationship with the caregiver**

Marie was speaking at an Alzheimer's family support group recently. A man there said that he visited his wife, who had advanced-stage Alzheimer's, nearly every day, even though she didn't recognize him. He learned early on, however, that she knew when he'd missed a day. She'd always say, "You didn't come yesterday."

- **The person may enjoy being visited, even if he doesn't recognize the individual who's visiting him**

Marie had another personal experience that led her to this conclusion. Ed had many visitors he didn't recognize. When these people were there he'd often hold hands with them—female or male—the whole time. And he'd have long, pleasant talks with them. It was perfectly obvious he was enjoying himself. One should pay attention and see if one's loved one is enjoying the visit. Again, that's what matters.

Daniel is the course director for a college class that pairs students in an art therapy experience with persons who have Alzheimer's disease. The students develop relationships with and empathy for those with the condition. It can be difficult for the students at first, because some of their partners do not remember them from week to week. However, once the students realize that the value of the experience lies in the joy they can offer people in the present moment and the improved quality of life that can result, the experience becomes meaningful to them.

- **The caregiver may feel gratified that he's given his loved one pleasure**

Although the main focus of interactions should be the person with Alzheimer's, a caregiver might find there's an unexpected benefit for him, too. He may initially feel hurt or frustrated that his loved one doesn't recognize him, but if that hurdle is surpassed and it's clear that the person with Alzheimer's enjoys the visit, the care partner will probably feel gratified that he is giving his loved one pleasure. Research has found that caregivers might remain in a good mood for some time after the visit.

It is difficult for people to accept the fact that their loved ones don't recognize them, and it may take a long time to reach such acceptance. Furthermore, some simply won't be able to achieve this, as hard as they may try, but if they can come to terms with the situation, their lives will most likely improve significantly. (Keep reading for more on this topic.)

- **The person may remain in a good mood long after the visit is over**

Recent research suggests that people with advanced Alzheimer's may continue to experience the emotional effects of happy or sad experiences for hours after an event has passed. This, in turn, might promote a positive or negative emotional tone, depending on the tone of the visit.

For instance, if a person living with Alzheimer's is visited by someone who is cheerful and smiling, who sings familiar songs to them, and who is completely present with them in a compassionate interaction, the positive emotional tone of this visit may last for several hours.

Conversely, if the person encounters a caregiver who is gruff, demanding ("Go and get your bath!"), or demeaning ("I'll have to get you a bib because you are spilling your food!") then the experience may cause a negative emotional reaction. Challenging behaviors may result and make the person more difficult to care for.

3. If the Person Finds a New Love

Beth was sitting in the nursing home room of her husband, Bernie, waiting for him to return from lunch. One can imagine her surprise when he walked in holding hands with a woman who lived in the facility. The pain was piercing, and she hardly knew how to react as the two sat down beside each other on the sofa, still holding hands. The pain was worse still when they smooched.

Let us say right up front that this is a controversial issue, and that some may find the suggestions the authors make objectionable, but the human need for relationships is ever present, even in those with Alzheimer's.

The care partner may have trouble accepting the fact that he's faced with this situation. He may feel betrayed by his loved one. The caregiver may feel angry and may even experience hatred toward the individual.

Perhaps the most well-known and admired person to find herself in this situation was Justice Sandra Day O'Connor. She retired from the Supreme Court to care for her husband, who had Alzheimer's.

According to a 2012 report in *USA Today* Mr. O'Conner found a new love. Although Justice O'Connor never commented publicly on the issue, her oldest son, Scott, did. According to the report, Scott compared his father to 'a teenager in love' and said, "For Mom to visit when he's happy…visiting with his girlfriend, sitting on the porch swing holding hands, was a relief after a painful period. She was thrilled that Dad was relaxed and happy."

Justice O'Connor is to be commended indeed for attaining this level of acceptance of a most difficult situation—something many spouses are never able to do.

It may take months or even years to come to accept this type of situation. Some may never accept it. That's certainly understandable, but if the caregiver can be content that his spouse is happy, he will be far less stressed and more pleased with his spouse and the spouse's new relationship.

4. If the Loved One Loses the Ability to Talk

If the person with Alzheimer's no longer talks, his caregiver may feel he can no longer communicate with that person. Again, one may feel it's the end of his relationship with the person, and that his loved one has lost a large part of his humanity and the ability to participate in life in a meaningful way. This may cut the care partner to the quick. He may not know what to do when he visits. He might simply sit in silence as though he, too, has lost the ability to talk.

Nothing could be further from the truth. There are several forms of nonverbal communication that can help reach the person living with Alzheimer's and continue the relationship, sometimes even on a deep level. Here are three of the most important ones:

- **Touch**

Using touch, such as described above in the case of Marie's interactions with Doris, is one way to communicate. Look at the person's face while holding hands or after hugging. Is he smiling? Does it look as though a connection is taking place?

There are many ways to use touch. These include, among many, holding hands, hugging, kissing, giving the person a gentle shoulder massage, or shaking hands. People in an advanced stage of the disease may enjoy having lotion applied to their hands. The caregiver should watch closely for any negative reactions his loved one may display and always ask if the person minds being touched, even if it isn't clear that the person can understand the question.

- **Smiling**

People with Alzheimer's tend to mirror the emotions of those around him. A smile is universally recognized as a gesture that conveys a positive emotion and regard. If the caregiver smiles, he may find that the person he's visiting will smile, too, indicating that that the individual with Alzheimer's may feel a positive emotion.

- **Visual cues**

Requests can be communicated through visual cues, such as pointing, touching, or handing a loved one an object he could or should use. For example, if the caregiver wants the person to drink some water, he can point to the glass or put a full glass near the person, and/or then pick it up and hand it to him.

5. If The Person Needs Hospice Care

This is the last of the five most difficult situations a caregiver may face. The need to involve hospice can be extremely difficult and even depressing. It's common to dwell on dark thoughts of impending death.

The very word 'hospice' can be frightening. This truly does signify that the end is near. One is about to lose his loved one, as difficult or wonderful as the relationship may be.

Some caregivers experience what is called 'anticipatory grief.' That is, they begin grieving over the person's death even before the individual dies. A care partner might want to consider getting counseling to help him cope. Most hospice organizations offer bereavement counseling programs for family members or friends.

Caregivers should keep in mind that their loved ones may not be aware that death is approaching. Conversely, people with Alzheimer's may, at some level, perceive that the end is near. Either way, the caregiver's suffering is real. But there is still the opportunity to have a relationship and to enjoy life with the loved one until the end. This will require an intentional acceptance, as well as gratitude for being given a life shared with the person.

Here's Marie's personal experience with finding a way to accept hospice care:

At first she was in denial. Even though Ed's medical team told her it was likely that Ed would pass away within six months, she continued believing and behaving as though he would live another year or two, or even more.

Marie eventually overcame her denial and decided to at least consider obtaining hospice care for Ed. However, she felt as though this would be tantamount to signing his death warrant. She knew that was ridiculous, but that's how she felt.

She delayed the call to hospice for weeks, telling herself Ed didn't need it quite yet. The truth was that Marie wasn't able to deal with it quite yet. Seeing how weak and frail Ed was, she finally felt compelled to take action. She consulted Dr. Doug Smucker, a family physician who specialized in end-of-life care.

After answering all of Marie's questions, Doug looked at her kindly and said, "You know, Marie, the real question for the caregiver is 'how can I help the person have the highest possible quality of life in the time that is remaining?'"

That completely changed Marie's thinking about the situation. It gave her a new and positive goal: to bring Ed as much happiness as possible. There was something she could do. It led her to think about all the special things she could do for Ed: visiting him more often, taking her little Shih Tzu to see him, having a classical violinist come and play a concert just for Ed in his room, reading to him from *The New York Times*, and buying Ed even more of the little stuffed animals he loved so much.

After that talk with Doug, Marie spent many pleasant hours thinking up special ways to bring Ed pleasure. Once she got her mind off his looming death, they were able to have a beautiful, pleasurable, months-long conclusion to their life together.

For Daniel's dad, the impending end became apparent when he had recurrent battles with pneumonia. His dad couldn't seem to recover from these infections and continued to aspirate, even on his own saliva (This is common in persons with end-stage Alzheimer's). This prompted the medical team to recommend hospice care as the most compassionate option.

Daniel's family, too, had some negative perceptions of hospice due to lack of knowledge. Fortunately, Daniel, a neurologist with experience in end-of-life care, was able to share his positive perceptions about hospice with the rest of the family. In addition, Daniel's father's attending physician served as the medical director of the hospice facility, assuring continuity of care.

From the moment Daniel's father entered the facility, the warmth and compassion of the staff embraced Daniel's father and his family. The place felt like home, with windows, fireplaces, bird feeders, music, quilts, and works of art. The staff was attentive to every need. Their goal was to make Daniel's dad as comfortable and cared for as possible.

This was not a place to die. This was a place to be comforted and honored for being a human being with innate dignity who was at the end of his earthly existence.

The family was no less embraced. Chaplains, social workers, nurses, and volunteers were available to guide the family through the process and answer questions. There was always food that had been brought in by various families, religious groups, and others. The quality of the experience made Daniel and his family strong advocates for hospice care.

A loving, comfortable end-of-life experience is certainly the main reason to place a loved one in hospice care. However, there are financial benefits, as well. Medicare and other insurers often will pay for services and medical supplies that are not otherwise covered.

In reality, the decision to enroll a loved one in hospice care signifies anything but giving up. The authors believe it is the most courageous, selfless, and compassionate action one can possibly take once a loved one once has reached the final stages of his disease.

Chapter 6: The Role of Grief on the Journey to Acceptance

<u>Loss</u>

Love and loss go hand in hand. When we lose something or someone vital and precious, we must give ourselves permission to grieve that loss to completion, or we will never be able to live fully again. The life cycle of grief brings love's bud to a flower. Love suffers and grows, or it isn't love at all. Everything else just suffers and dies. Love lives on through the loss.

Daniel

When Ed was first diagnosed with Alzheimer's, Marie was devastated. She knew in her heart she'd never be able to accept the situation. It was so bad she couldn't even have a meaningful conversation with him. He couldn't praise her for her accomplishments. He couldn't give her advice about her problems. He couldn't be that rock who had always been there for her. Marie was lost, deep in the clutches of grief.

Then one day on a whim and against her better judgment, Marie took Ed a little stuffed animal. He loved it. They started playing simple games with it. It was fun. It was like a mother playing with her young child, so Marie took him more little stuffed animals. He loved each one more than the one before.

After a few weeks, Marie realized that her heart had changed forever. She had finally found a way to relate to Ed—one that was satisfying for both of them. She was delighted to see his happiness. When she realized she could bring pleasure to her 'new Ed,' it was more than enough to make up for the loss of their previous relationship.

Make no mistake about it—this state of acceptance will not be easy to achieve. It will take time, and the amount of time will vary from person to person. It could take weeks, months, or even years. In the beginning, some are convinced they won't be able to do it. In fact, despite how hard they try, some people never reach a state of acceptance.

Grief probably needs to come before acceptance. It's necessary to grieve the loss of the mental image of a loved one as he used to be. Grief for the fact that the person isn't ever going to get better. Grief because the person will continue deteriorating over time. One may feel overwhelmed by grief.

If the person living with Alzheimer's is placed in a care facility, most of his needs may be met by the staff. The family caregiver may feel unneeded. When one cares for someone for a long time and then that person doesn't seem to need the caregiver anymore, there is such an enormous vacuum that the caregiver may feel useless and depressed.

One may even feel he has let the person down, that he is not 'good enough' to care for the person at home, that he has done the worst thing possible, that he is a total failure. The caregiver may worry that other people think badly of him and are criticizing him behind his back.

Caregivers will probably miss having their loved ones around all day every day. No matter how relieved they may feel that they are no longer on duty 24/7, caregivers may still feel deep grief at the loss of companionship, no matter how difficult it was to keep their loved one at home.

The caregiver also may feel angry at his loved one for changing. He may feel angry if he can no longer have meaningful conversations with the person who has Alzheimer's. If that person doesn't recognize the caregiver anymore, the caregiver may feel even more anger. He may feel so angry that he doesn't want to visit the person. He may even wish the person were dead. This, too, is normal. Anger is part of the grieving process.

It's important to take time to grieve. To be gentle with oneself. The grief will probably end sooner or later, and the caregiver may finally be free to accept the situation, which will lead to the possibility of truly enjoying his relationship with the person and having joyous visits.

Chapter 7: Make Peace with God

<u>Control</u>

Control is an illusion I sought for years. I now feel peace in knowing I control nothing, God controls everything, and God is Love.

Daniel

"If there is a God, why would he/she do this to my loved one? I don't deserve this. Life is so cruel and unfair."

How many people have heard Alzheimer's caregivers say something such as the statement above? How many have said this to themselves or at least thought it?

The age-old question, "Why do bad things happen to good people?" is certainly relevant to making peace with God.

Trying to answer this question is beyond the scope of this book. Furthermore, the authors don't presume to be qualified to do justice to this issue, but they do know from experience that resentment in general, and against God in particular, can poison one's caregiving journey. As Malachy McCourt once said,

"Resentment is like taking poison and waiting for the other person to die."

Facing the Herculean challenges of caregiving requires all the strength that can be mustered, including spiritual strength. It has been the authors' experience that caregivers who develop what the authors call 'spiritual intentionality' are better able to face these challenges and retain their joy and hope than those who seek to go it alone, fueled by denial, anger and resentment.

Resentment and anger are most often directed toward God, whether or not this is recognized and acknowledged. These attitudes can be exhausting and can make a caregiver feel all alone to carry the 'weight of the world.'

Spiritual intentionality in caregiving means cultivating the capacity to give meaning to suffering; to see problems and challenges that confront one and his loved one as opportunities for growth, transformation, and greater expression of love in the act of caring for another.

This process is just that: a process, and it is not necessarily intuitive. It is certainly not easy, and it takes commitment, but as has been previously stated, it must begin with letting go, with realizing one is not in control of the circumstances. The caregiver can choose how he will respond to the person with Alzheimer's. Will resentment and anger rule the day, or will there be peace, serenity, and love?

It is obvious which would be the healthier of the two options, for both the caregiver and his loved one, and the process should be one of both giving and receiving. Those who only give and are not open to receive energy, presence, and love from people with Alzheimer's often experience burn out.

One may not be 'spiritual' or religious. However, the bottom line is that the road will be much smoother, and the capacity to experience joy in relationship with one's loved one will be much greater if the caregiver can acknowledge that he needs help.

Dr. James Houston, Professor of Spiritual Theology at Regent College in Vancouver, BC and a caregiver himself, said the following to Daniel in a recent interview: "The pain that is brought into God's presence enriches us for the rest of our lives, but the pain that is borne in self-reliance and in a stoic fashion, repressing all emotion, brings death. In faith, we have the wonderful knowledge that we are never carrying the pain of caregiving on our own."

The question to be asked is not "Why do bad things happen to good people?" but "How do we and the ones we care for make the most of the present situation, grow in the process, and live as joyfully, peacefully, and lovingly as possible?" The authors assert that to do this one must make peace with God and learn to put away resentment.

Part II: Tips for Interacting With People Who Have Alzheimer's

Chapter 8: Tips for Interacting

<u>Love</u>

We who are care partners for those with Alzheimer's disease and other dementias must identify and embrace the love present within each individual, and we must enable the expression of that love for personhood to be preserved, and dignity promoted. We must also be fully cognizant of the love within ourselves and we must be willing to let it blossom vitally and beautifully in its melding together with that of another.

Daniel

Many people simply don't know how to interact with or entertain people who have Alzheimer's. The following tips will help you improve the quality of your relationship and visits. After a little thought and experience, you may come up with more tips yourself.

These tips are loosely organized in four groups: Nonverbal, Verbal, Things to Do (including Art, Music, Poetry, Movement, Pets, Children, and 'Props'), and Other Tips.

Nonverbal Tips:

1. **Make Eye Contact:** Always approach people with Alzheimer's face to face and make eye contact. It is vital that they see you. Otherwise, they may not realize you're there or that you're talking to them.

2. **Be at Their Level:** Move your head to be at the same level as theirs. You may need to kneel or sit down to accomplish this. Do not stand or hover over them. It may feel intimidating.

3. **Don't Talk to Them From Behind:** This goes along with tip number 1. You can't make eye contact if you are behind people. In addition, if you're behind them, they may not be able to hear or understand you. Additionally, it could startle a person into having a violent reaction.

4. **Smile Frequently:** Smile if you're telling a humorous story or if your loved one is telling you one. Also, smile if one of you is talking about something pleasant. Research has shown that smiling at a person can cause that person to feel better and smile back.

5. **Don't Make Sudden Movements:** If you make sudden movements, it can scare a person with Alzheimer's. For example, move slowly when you are getting up from your chair to leave.

6. **Shake Hands:** Consider shaking hands at the beginning of each visit. This is one form of therapeutic touch (tip 10). Put your hand out and see

if the person you're visiting grasps it. If not, then you can lower your hand and forget about it.

7. **Use Visual Cues:** Point to, touch, or hand your loved one the item you want him to use. For example, if you want him to sit down, point to the chair and sit down yourself.

8. **Don't Sit With Your Arms Crossed:** This advice is the same for interacting with someone with Alzheimer's as it is for interacting with someone who does not have the disease. This pose tends to convey anger and/or a closed mind.

9. **Sit With Your Palms Turned Upward:** This pose says, "I'm receptive to you."

10. **Use Therapeutic Touch:** Try hugging the person, kissing him on the cheek, giving him a gentle shoulder massage, holding hands, or putting your arm around him.

11. **Take a Blanket, Quilt, or Shawl:** Wrapping up in a blanket or shawl may be especially appealing to people in the later stages of Alzheimer's.

12. **Laugh a Lot:** Sometimes laughter is the best medicine. It will lift the mood of both the person with Alzheimer's and you. So be sure you arrive for visits with a supply of simple jokes or funny stories.

Verbal Tips:

13. **Say What You Are Going to Do Before You Do It:** This is particularly important if you are going to touch someone so they don't think you are grabbing them.

14. **Speak Slowly:** Speak at about half your normal speed. Take a breath between each sentence. Give the person a chance to catch up with your words. Otherwise, your words may be received as blurry noise with no clear meaning.

15. **Don't Be Condescending:** Don't talk to people with Alzheimer's as though they're children. It's easy to 'baby-talk' to a person who has Alzheimer's, but if he doesn't understand you when you talk in a normal tone of voice he probably won't comprehend the 'baby-talk' either. Furthermore, this can feel degrading to a person with the disease, and may cause him to feel bad.

16. **Speak in Short Sentences:** Speak in short, direct sentences with only one idea to each sentence. Usually people with Alzheimer's can only focus on one idea at a time. If you speak in long sentences they may not be able to follow you, and they may just give up trying to talk with you at all.

17. **Ask Only One Question at a Time:** Let the person answer a question before you ask another. If you ask two or more questions at once, he probably won't be

able to remember them all. Again, the person may just give up trying to converse.

18. **Don't Ask "Do You Remember?"** Many times people with Alzheimer's will not be able to remember, and you are just pointing out their shortcomings. That may be perceived as insulting and can cause them to feel anger and/or embarrassment. For example, instead of saying, "Do you remember that we played checkers the last time I was here?" say "We played checkers the last time I was here, and it was fun."

19. **Turn Negatives Into Positives:** For example, say, "Let's laugh" instead of "Don't be so serious." Or "Let's do this" instead of "Don't do that."

20. **Validate Feelings:** Don't try to convince people with Alzheimer's that they shouldn't be feeling a certain way, especially if they are sad or upset about something. It's tempting to try to convince them they should not be upset, but it's better to say something such as, "I see that you are angry (sad, upset, etc.) Tell me about it." Be empathic and let them talk about their feelings. After that, say something reassuring. Then change the subject to something pleasant.

21. **Talk About Old Times More Than Recent Ones:** The person is more likely to remember events from his distant past, so you might ask him to tell you about his high school or college days. Then try to tie the positive reminiscences to the present. For example,

"You have told me that you loved the biscuits your mother used to make for you when you were a child. I have heard they have wonderful biscuits here, as well. I can't wait to try them with you." This can anchor pleasant memories in the present moment, fostering a positive emotional tone and validating the person with dementia in his current state of being.

22. **What to Do When Someone Keeps Repeating the Same Question:** Answer the question patiently as though it's the first time they asked it, because for them it is. They can't remember they already asked the question. This will require patience on your part, but will be well worth the effort. After answering the question, you can try to redirect the conversation, but it may not work.

23. **What to Do When Someone Keeps Repeating the Same Story:** Respond as though it's the first time they told you the story. They can't remember they just told it to you. This will have the same positive consequences as following tip number 22. Also, as with tip number 22, you can try to redirect the conversation after they are finished telling the story.

24. **If the Person Starts Getting Agitated, Stop What You're Talking About:** If you quickly change the subject, he will probably forget all about the previous, upsetting topic.

25. **Do Not Correct the Person:** This may embarrass him or lead to an argument. For example, if he says it's Christmas time when it isn't, just let it go. It isn't

really important that he know what season it is. Don't try to drag the person into your reality. Meet him in his.

26. **Do Not Argue:** Don't even think about arguing with a person who has Alzheimer's. You can't win. Again, the issue you're tempted to argue about probably isn't important.

27. **Use Their Name Frequently:** Most people respond positively to hearing their name, and people with Alzheimer's are usually no different.

28. **Don't Tell People in the Later Stages of the Disease That a Loved One Has Passed Away:** This may just upset them. It's best to say something such as "He's away and will return soon." Then change the subject. Another approach is to comment, "You must be thinking about that person. Tell me about him." However, you can tell people in the early stages of the condition about a loved one's death, but don't belabor the information.

29. **Don't Even Bring up Topics That May Upset Them:** This may lead to a nasty argument, so if you don't generally agree about politics or religion, just don't bring them up.

30. **Types of Questions to Avoid:** To avoid confusing or embarrassing a person with Alzheimer's, don't ask questions beginning with 'who,' 'what,' 'where' or 'when.' He probably won't remember these details. For example, if he just returned from a field trip ask,

"Did you enjoy your trip?" not "Where did you go on your trip?" (This assumes they remember the trip.) Also, avoid questions starting with 'how' or 'why.' The answers may be too complicated. If you ask, "How did you find your wallet?" he may not even remember he lost his wallet. It's better to say, "I see you found your wallet. You must be happy about that."

Things to Do (Including Art, Music, Poetry, Movement, Pets, Children, and 'Props')

31. **Do Something Interactive:** Take 'props' (such as items related to one of the person's special interests) to bring up pleasant memories and serve as a focal point for interacting. For example, bring a woman's wedding dress, or if she was an accountant, take a calculator and let her use it.

32. **Take a Pet:** Persons with Alzheimer's often respond to pets more than they respond to people. If possible, take the same kind of pet they had previously. So, take a dog to dog lovers; a cat to those who loved cats. You can even take a bird in a cage to a visit.

33. **Take a Child:** As with pets, infants and children may reach a person with Alzheimer's on a deep level. Try taking an infant or young child with you to visit. Ideally, take no more than one at a time. Let your loved one hold the infant (if you're sure he can safely do so), and arrange for simple games through which

he can engage with the child. (Make sure the child feels comfortable with the interaction.)

34. **Take Art Supplies:** Art involves parts of the brain different from the areas that control language and other cognitive processes that are being destroyed by the disease. Creating art gives people a way to express themselves, especially when verbal abilities are failing. This may be helpful even with people who never did any kind of artwork before developing Alzheimer's.

35. **Go on a Visit to an Art Museum:** If you can still take your loved one out in public, try going to an art museum. Research has shown that just looking at art can be beneficial. Another possibility would be to take him to an art fair.

36. **Play Music:** Music also uses many different parts of the brain. Play the type of music they liked before they developed Alzheimer's. For example, don't play Rock for people who were classical music lovers. Dan Cohen, a social worker from New York, created the Music and Memory Foundation based on his experience with personalized iPod playlists and their profound positive effects on people with dementia. If you don't know what kind of music they like, music that was popular during their teenage years and their twenties is usually a good choice.

37. **Bring a Small Wrapped Gift:** Wrap the gift no matter how insignificant it is. The person will probably enjoy ripping off the wrapping paper as

much or even more than actually having the gift. Don't feel badly if the gift is put aside immediately and subsequently ignored. He may forget you even gave him a gift. The important thing is that he enjoyed receiving it.

38. **Take Them to a Memory Cafe:** Memory cafes give people with Alzheimer's the opportunity to relax and interact with others who have dementia, something that most people with the condition enjoy.

39. **Arrange for Musicians to Perform:** This provides more stimulation than simply listening to a CD, iPod, or radio. You can do this in the person's room at a facility as easily as you can do it at home if that's where he's living.

40. **Play Background Music:** Play soft, soothing background music unless you can see that it's distracting the person. If it is, then stop it. Watch his face carefully to determine if you should stop.

41. **Have a Sing-Along:** Sing-alongs give people with Alzheimer's a chance to actively participate in musical experiences. Many people with the disease can sing the words of a song even if they can't remember other things. If you're at home and you don't play an instrument to accompany the music, you can sing without one, or you might sing to recorded music.

42. **Avoid These Types of Music:** Avoid music that is sad, frenetic, or dissonant. This may upset the person or make him agitated.

43. **If They Played an Instrument, Give it to Them:** They may still be able to play and may enjoy it very much. Even if they can't play it, they may derive pleasure from simply holding the instrument.

44. **Give Them Rhythmic, Percussive Musical Instruments:** Give them instruments, such as drums or tambourines they may play while listening to live or recorded music. This allows them to actively participate in a music experience through keeping time with or moving to the rhythm of the song. This can be enjoyed even by those in the later stages of the disease. Try moving with them.

45. **Recite Familiar Things:** Try reciting poems to or with the person. Select poems he will recognize. You might also read from the Bible (if the person was religious), long-loved novels, or other material if the person was a life-long reader. Even those in the latest stages will find your voice comforting, regardless of whether or not they recognize what you're reciting.

46. **Write Poetry With the Person:** Write simple poems and ask the person to help you by adding lines. It's his participation that matters, not how good the poems are.

47. **Play Simple Games:** People with Alzheimer's may be able to play games they liked before developing Alzheimer's, but you may need to simplify the games. (Playing catch with a small ball gave Daniel's dad

much enjoyment, even very late into the disease's progression.)

48. **Work on Jigsaw Puzzles:** The person may enjoy doing jigsaw puzzles. Keep in mind you may have to use puzzles with fewer and larger pieces. (Go to puzzlestoremember.org to find these.)

49. **Look at Old Photographs:** This can help people remember events of the past, which can be pleasurable for them. Take a picture album to thumb through and/or hang photographs in a collage on their wall.

50. **Watch Old Movies or TV Shows:** People with Alzheimer's may enjoy watching movies or television shows they previously liked. Try to avoid movies and shows that are sad or have complicated plots. Musicals or comedy programs they may have enjoyed watching in earlier years are particularly good choices.

51. **Try Giving Them Dolls or Stuffed Animals:** These items may reach people with Alzheimer's on a level we cannot. It seems that they often feel the dolls or stuffed animals are real and enjoy cuddling with them and/or taking care of them.

Other Tips

52. **Knock Before Entering Their Room:** Knock on the door and ask for permission to come in. You certainly wouldn't want someone to barge in on you

when you have your door closed, and people with Alzheimer's are no different.

53. **Step out When He Is Receiving Personal Care:** If the person lives in a facility, allow him to retain his sense of modesty and dignity by temporarily leaving the room if he is being changed or receiving other personal care.

54. **Don't Visit if They Already Have a Visitor:** If a person already has one or more visitors, adding another one may create too much stimulation for him. It's best to leave and come back later. Similarly, when you go to visit it would be best not to take more than one other person with you. Furthermore, if you bring another person, don't spend the time talking to each other. Do your 'catching up' later. Finally, if someone you know is coming to visit the person, it's best to ask them to come alone.

55. **Keep Visiting Even Though The Person May Not Remember Who You Are:** Even though your loved one may not recognize you, he may enjoy visiting with you, and that's what matters. You may gently remind him of who you are and how you're related to him, but if he doesn't seem to understand, then just drop it and enjoy the visit. Recent studies suggest that even people in the later stages of Alzheimer's are affected by the emotional content of a visit for a period of time after it, even if they have forgotten the visit itself.

Conclusion: Putting these tips into practice will not only make your visits go more smoothly, but also will increase the chances of creating joy for you and for your loved one.

Note: Some of these tips are from the following sources: an article by Carole Larkin, an interview with Tom and Karen Brenner, an interview with Teepa Snow, the Alzheimer's Association website, and an article by Bob DeMarco. (Refer to the Appendix for citations of these works.)

Chapter 9: How to Behave When Visiting in a Facility

Visiting a loved one in an assisted living, long-term care, hospice, or other type of facility is essential for your well-being as well as his. When the person is admitted, talk with the administrator or director of nursing about the facility's policies for visits. Some have written guidelines. If they don't, have a general discussion with the official about the topic.

There may be some unwritten rules: do's and don'ts regarding your interactions with the residents and staff. Some of the more important ones are summarized below.

'Don'ts' for Visiting Your Loved One:

Don't take unruly pets or undisciplined children to visit. If children are well behaved, however, they can provide extra pleasure to your loved one. Take a pet if your loved one enjoys it, but check with the facility first to find out if it has a policy about pet visits. Some facilities require proof the animal's shots are up-to-date.

Don't wake up residents who are sleeping. They probably need the sleep and won't enjoy your visit if they are groggy.

Don't take food or beverages your loved one isn't allowed to have. Check with the staff first if you have any questions about what's permissible. Also, never give food to other residents without checking with the staff.

Don't stay too long. It may tire your loved one and interfere with the staff's provision of needed care. How long is too long? That depends. It's different for every resident. Look for cues that your loved one may be getting tired or stressed out.

Do not interrupt the resident's activity time. Find out from the staff when activities are scheduled. It may be acceptable to sit beside him and just observe unless your presence distracts him from the activity. You can get guidance from the staff.

'Do's' for Interacting With Staff:

Learn the names of staff members involved in your loved one's care and be warm in your interactions with them. Thank them for any special services. Also, be sure to show respect for non-caregivers, such as the dietary or laundry service staff members.

If the facility has visiting hours, respect them. Otherwise, you may impede the staff from carrying out their caregiving duties.

Keep the lines of communication open. Should there be a serious problem, communicate it promptly and directly to the administrator or director of nursing. Never confront an aide or nurse directly.

Attend the regularly scheduled care conferences to which you are invited. This is a good time to discuss your wishes or concerns about the care your loved one is receiving and get updates on how he is doing.

'Don'ts':

Don't order the staff around. Ask the administrator to whom you should address any special requests for the nurses or aides.

Don't give monetary tips or bring gifts for the staff if the facility has guidelines forbidding them. Some institutions allow holiday gifts. If gifts are not allowed, give handwritten thank you cards to the people you want to recognize.

Don't be a chronic complainer. It's like crying wolf. Before you lodge a complaint, ask yourself if there's really a problem or it's just a matter of personal preference. If it's the latter, it's best to just let it go.

Don't have unrealistic expectations. Understand that staff members have many patients to care for and may not have time to do every tiny thing you'd like. Again, before complaining, make sure there's a problem.

Don't visit at mealtime unless you have checked with the administrator regarding the facility's policies. Some nursing homes welcome visitors to dine with their loved ones; others do not.

Don't take out your own guilt on the staff. Ask yourself whether the issue is real, or whether it's your own guilt talking.

Following these simple guidelines will help you avoid problems. It will also make your visits far more pleasant for everyone.

Note: This chapter incorporates some tips mentioned to Marie in an interview with Susan Gilster, PhD, executive director of the

Gilster Group, an organization that transforms memory care, person-centered care, and cultures.

PART III: Stories About Our Personal Joyous Relationships and Visits

Chapter 10: Meet Ed and Meet Marie's 'Ladies'

Before presenting our personal stories, we introduce you to our loved ones (in Chapters 10 and 11.)

Meet Edward Theodoru, PhD: Marie's Romanian Life Partner

Early Life

Ed was born and raised in Bucharest, Romania. He became a defense attorney and had exceptional professional success. In the mid '60s, after ten years of petitioning the 'damned communist regime' (as he called it), begging them to let him leave the country, he was finally granted permission to go.

When he arrived in the US, at first he worked at menial jobs while pursuing a doctorate in Romance Languages and Literatures at the University of Cincinnati. After that, he became a professor of French at the nearby Northern Kentucky University (NKU), while also teaching French at the University of Cincinnati's Evening College.

Chivalrous Despite Alzheimer's

Ed was the consummate old-school European gentleman. He routinely kissed the hands of ladies to whom he was introduced, pulled out their chairs in restaurants, and opened doors for them.

In addition, he sent flowers for any occasion (or even no occasion) and delivered a constant stream of sincere compliments. On my birthday he always snuck into my house and left a vase of yellow roses on my dining room table. It made me feel so special.

One might expect that he'd lose these gentlemanly qualities when he developed Alzheimer's but, if anything, he became more chivalrous. For example, he always held the hands of his visitors the entire time they were there.

He thanked each staff member profusely for anything they did for him or even just for stopping by to say hello. He not only thanked them, he told them how beautiful they were and that he was so lucky to have their help. He then asked them when they were coming back and exclaimed, "Marvelous" no matter what they answered.

One day when I was signing out at the desk, the receptionist on duty told me that Ed must have been quite the ladies' man in his time.

She said he had come up to her desk the previous evening and told her, "You're the most beautiful woman in the world, and I really mean it from my heart; it's not just words from my lips."

Every time I visited Ed at the Alois Alzheimer Center where he was living, he told me how beautiful I was. At one point, I started getting a little tired of it, so I asked him if he could please stop telling me that.

He answered, "I can…but it will be difficult."

Then there was a long silence, which he finally broke by asking, "Can I tell you how beautiful your earrings are?" We both burst into laughter.

That Stunning Theodoru Memory and Intellect

Going back now to the time before he developed Alzheimer's, Ed was a true Renaissance man, and his memory, in particular, had been astonishing. Anything he read, heard, or saw went into it and never left. It was that simple. Ed also knew seven languages. We often say such people are walking encyclopedias. Ed was so much more. He was a walking library.

He'd received a classic European education in Bucharest, had studied further in France and the US, and had read nearly all the 1,200 books in his personal library "plus," as he once said to a friend who was admiring his collection, "a few more." The 'few more' were, in fact, 'hunnerds' if not 'tousands' more.

The Bad Typewriter

Ed's quirky accent and idiosyncratic use of the English language was sometimes amusing. Although his vocabulary was rich and sophisticated—certainly more so than mine—he did make some rather endearing mistakes at times. For example, he once informed a woman who was interviewing him for a job that he was 'a bad typewriter.'

"Go get a chopstick from my medicine cabinet," he told me once when my lips were chapped.

One time while in the car I needed a Kleenex. He told me, "Look in the glove department."

Ed was a horrible driver and often asked me why other cars were 'horning' at him. He was always returning shoes because "they hurt my feet fingers."

But my favorite by far was when he asked a clerk at Walgreen's, "Do you have any hangovers?"

She looked shocked and asked, "What?"

He said, "Hangovers. Do you have any hangovers?"

Well, he wanted clip-on sunglasses. You know…they 'hang over' your regular glasses. Needless to say, the clerk was taken aback.

Ed also had a heavy accent. For one thing, he couldn't pronounce 'th.' That made for a rather interesting name change for his friend Henry Sexton III, whom he always innocently called Henry Sexton 'the turd.' Try as I might, I could never teach him how to pronounce 'third.'

Finally, displaying an outsider's insight into the English language, Ed asked me once, "Why do you say in English 'I'm pissed off?' It would be more proper to say, 'I feel pissed on.'" We both laughed, and I had to agree with him.

Our Relationship

I often think about how Ed had boldly tricked me into going on a first date with him without me even knowing it was a date. I was a lowly graduate student of musicology at the time. The phone jarred me awake from a pleasant Saturday afternoon's much-needed nap a few weeks after Guido, my Italian history professor and boyfriend, had introduced me to Ed at the university.

I lifted the receiver and said, "Hello."

"Is this Ma-r-r-ie?" Ed asked in his heavily accented voice.

"Yes, it is."

The booming voice then said, "Here is Edward Theodoru."

I was thoroughly confused. I couldn't imagine any reason for Ed to be calling me, but after some awkward initial niceties I found out the true reason for his call.

"Would you have 'dee-ner' with me this evening?" he asked.

Then I was even more baffled. He knew I was deeply in love with Guido, his friend and colleague. I couldn't believe he had the audacity to make a play for me, so I just stood there, not yet fully awake and too confused to know how to respond.

"Ask a girlfriend to come with you," Ed told me, evidently noting my indecision. He sounded so innocent and sincere.

Well, that changed everything. If I could bring a friend, then he obviously wasn't intending this as a date. He probably just wanted some company for 'dee-ner'. I accepted and—just as this little trickster had hoped—I didn't bother asking a girlfriend to come along. That's how naïve I was.

I was twenty-five and decidedly immature for my age. I didn't know how old he was. He was certainly more than old enough to be my father, but then so was Guido, so I didn't really think much about it. Besides, this wasn't a date, so our relative ages didn't matter.

Ed lived at the Edgecliff apartment building near Eden Park, which just happened to have a restaurant, and he just happened to suggest we go there for 'dee-ner.' In my youthful innocence, I never saw it coming.

Soon after we were seated, a rather young-looking teenaged waiter wearing a black shirt and tight black pants, brought us glasses of ice water with lemon.

A little later, we were interrupted by the waiter, who arrived and put down our plates. After asking us if we needed anything else—we said we didn't—the waiter left.

The moment he was out of ear shot, Ed casually asked me in his deep bass voice, "Would you like to go to 'Ee-taly' with me on a vacation sometime?"

Oops! I guess I was wrong about his intent for that 'dee-ner.' It was a date, after all.

I just stared at him. I had no idea what to say. I tried to think of an answer. Finally one came to me.

"I'll have to think about it," I said.

We soon fell in love and had a whirlwind romance. I was ecstatic, but after around three years we began having bad and frequent arguments. Finally, I couldn't take it anymore, so I ended the relationship. Or so I thought. Turned out that that we soon became friends. Then best friends. Then life partners—soul mates, really—in a loving relationship that would last until the very end.

Alzheimer's Strikes

In the year 2000, Ed began showing clear signs of dementia. I was in denial for months, but finally couldn't ignore it any longer.

The first dramatic event happened one evening in January, 2005. I did all of Ed's grocery shopping for him, and when I suggested that I pick up some specific items for him at Kroger's, he didn't recognize several of his favorite foods. He didn't even remember Starbucks, which was the only coffee he had used for years.

I mentioned to him that he should put the coffee in the freezer (as he always did), and he asked me where the freezer was. When I told him it was in the kitchen, he didn't remember what a kitchen was.

"Kitchen," he asked. "What's a kitchen? I don't have a kitchen."

Alarmed, I tried to jog his memory.

"You know, where your stove is."

"My stove? What is a stove? Do I have a stove?"

I continued, "Yes, where you cook your food." That didn't help either.

He called me back a little later. He said that he had found his kitchen, but that there were only clothes and shoes in it.

Ed's symptoms progressed slowly over the years. Beginning in June of 2005, I started keeping detailed records of his symptoms to show his physician. The entries included, among many others, the following:

June 1: Ed has always taken great pride in his appearance, but came to the door to receive expected guests when he did not have his dentures in. The most amazing thing was that he didn't even seem to know or care.

June 3: He couldn't remember how to operate his TV. Didn't know what the remote was.

June 10: Ed called me to ask what his phone number was, even though he'd had the number for 40 years.

June 12: He couldn't remember where he kept important items including, unbelievably, his clothes.

June 15: Ed was terribly distressed because he couldn't find his slacks, which were on the bed right beside him.

As you may imagine, it only got worse as time went by.

The Alois Alzheimer Center

After witnessing many more clear signs of Alzheimer's, as well as numerous falls, I realized that Ed could no longer live alone. I made arrangements for him to move to Cincinnati's wonderful Alois Alzheimer Center. But then the strangest thing happened: he changed his mind and refused to go.

For three solid months I begged him to go. I cried about it and implored him to go. I harassed him about it. I talked to him about it in reasonable terms. I even threatened him about it. It seemed it was the only thing we ever talked about. All to no avail.

Every single time his response was the same: "I'd rather die than move there."

Finally, one day when I told him for the hundredth time that he'd be much better off at the Alois Center, he glared at me and asked, "Who's keeping me from moving there?"

It had finally happened. His dementia was so advanced that he didn't remember his opposition to moving. I hurriedly packed a bag and took him there the next day before he could change his mind again. Once at the Center, he adjusted well and spent a wonderful 17 months there.

Come Back Early Today

I'd been visiting Ed only on Sundays because I was preoccupied with my professional duties and an upcoming job interview. I just didn't have time to visit more often, but one day I decided to go see him, although it was only Saturday.

When I arrived, I found him in bed asleep.

They must have let him skip breakfast, I thought.

He was lying on his back with his mouth open. His beige blanket was pulled up under his chin, covering every square inch of him except his head. He was often asleep when I arrived, but usually I was able to awaken him and get him out of bed for a lively visit. So I called out his name. He opened his eyes then looked over at the housekeeper who was silently mopping the floor.

"Isn't she beautiful?" he said, referring to me.

Mary smiled and nodded.

I walked over to his bed and handed him the large white teddy bear with curly fur I'd gotten for him at Walgreen's. Never tiring of receiving new stuffed animals, he took it in his arms and smiled like a four-year-old who came downstairs on Christmas morning to discover a huge pile of presents under the tree.

He hugged the bear to his chest, caressed it, and kissed it several times.

"Do you like it?" I asked.

"Like it? I'm overcome with affection for him."

"Do you want to get up?" I asked.

"Sleepy!" he called out loudly in a child-like voice.

I sat down on the bed and held his hand. We hadn't held hands since we were intimately involved all those many years before, but I felt like holding his hand that day. He dozed intermittently, looking so frail.

His breathing was strange. I'd never seen him breathe like that. He took several short breaths—huffing and puffing like someone who'd just run up several flights of stairs—then he stopped breathing completely for several seconds. Each time he stopped breathing I watched his chest intently, waiting to make sure it started moving again.

This is how it will end someday, I thought. He will be dozing like this and breathing like this, and stopping to breathe like this, and simply not take another breath.

We talked in between his intermittent dozing. Nothing important. We talked about whether he had breakfast that day, he told me how beautiful I was, and he talked about having seen his father—who was long deceased—the night before.

"I have to go home now," I said after a while. I let go of his hand reluctantly and got up to put on my coat.

"When are you coming back?"

"Tomorrow," I answered as always, getting my gloves from my purse.

Even though I wasn't planning to go back the following day, I said it to make him happy. I knew he'd never know the difference

But instead of saying, "Marvelous!" as he did every time, he suddenly looked disappointed, as though I'd said I wasn't coming back for a month.

"Tomorrow?" he asked. "What do you have to do that's so important you can't come back until tomorrow?"

I didn't know what to say.

"Well, when do you want me to come back?" I finally asked.

"Today!"

"Okay," I said, playing along. "I'll come back today."

"Early today!" he added firmly.

"Yes," I said. "I'll come back early today!"

"Marvelous!" he said.

He smiled, obviously convinced by my statement. He kissed my hand, and when I left I turned and blew kisses to him and he blew kisses back to me.

Had I Googled his breathing pattern, I would have realized the end was near, but I didn't Google it.

I awakened at 5:30 the next morning. Soon after, the jingling of my cell phone startled me. I picked it up. Caller ID said it was the Alois Center. I wondered why on earth they were calling me so early on a Sunday morning.

I flipped open the phone.

"Hello," I said.

"Hello, is this Marie Marley?" asked a woman whose voice I didn't recognize.

"Yes, it is," I answered.

"This is Joyce, from the Alois Center. I'm afraid I have bad news for you."

Oh my God. Ed's fallen and broken a hip, I thought.

But she said simply, "Edward is gone."

And thus ended a beautiful 30-year love story.

Author's Note: All of the stories about Ed are presented in greater detail in my book, *Come Back Early Today: A Memoir of Love, Alzheimer's and Joy* (available on Amazon).

Meet Marie's 'Ladies'

I took an early retirement from my job as a grant writer at the American Academy of Family Physicians in 2013 to devote myself entirely to my Alzheimer's work. That consists of blogging on the *Huffington Post*, the Alzheimer's Reading room, and Maria Shriver's website, as well as doing public speaking on Alzheimer's caregiving issues at support groups and professional meetings.

One day I was talking to my dogs' veterinarian, Ann McHugh, DVM. She told me she was volunteering to visit patients at a local hospice, and that it was very rewarding. This conversation eventually led to my decision to volunteer to visit some ladies with dementia at Brookdale Senior Living's Clare Bridge memory care facility in Overland Park, Kansas.

At first, I was quite concerned that visiting these ladies would remind me of Ed and make me sad. On the contrary, it has turned out to be a marvelous experience. I had always heard people say that volunteering gives them so much more than they receive. I didn't really believe it, but it is true. No matter what kind of mood I'm in when I arrive, I always feel happier when I leave.

Clare Bridge is an excellent place. First of all, it's a beautiful facility. Always sparkling clean and completely without odor, all of the rooms are spacious and in perfect condition. Some of the rooms even have kitchenettes, without, of course, potentially dangerous stoves or microwaves. There are under-the-counter refrigerators, small sinks, and many cabinets in which to store all manner of belongings.

More important than the appearance of the place, is that it provides an abundance of interesting, engaging activities for the residents.

Not only are there seemingly unending activities throughout the day, but also the residents are frequently taken out for drives, usually punctuated by lunch and/or ice cream.

It isn't unusual for me to arrive to visit and find all of 'My Ladies' carefully descending from the little bus that has taken them out. They may not remember the trip an hour later, but they typically remain in a good mood for a long time.

Furthermore, the nurses, aides, activity people, and all the rest of the staff are truly marvelous. Everyone is well-trained in how to communicate and interact with people who have dementia. Redirection comes so easily to them. Calming agitated residents is natural for them. Open displays of affection are often seen. As a matter of fact, this facility and its staff are so impressive that if I ever get Alzheimer's I'd like to live there myself!

I have visited seven ladies in all, usually three to four each time I go. One moved to another facility, and two have passed away, so I was assigned some new residents to visit, leaving me with three at present. They are in various stages of the illness.

On Christmas day last year, I spontaneously decided to go visit, even though I assumed most of 'My Ladies' would be at home with their families. I was quite surprised to find all of them in their rooms. I felt sad that they were alone on Christmas day, but was happy I was able to cheer them up.

Note: I have changed 'My Ladies' names and any clearly identifying information in the descriptions below to protect their privacy.

Nancy

Nancy, who didn't want to visit with me, was in the mid stage of Alzheimer's. The staff said she loved Elvis, so I bought an Elvis CD and played it for her. But instead of enjoying it, she became very sad and began to cry.

"It's so beautiful it makes me cry," she said.

During the few weeks I did visit her, she often told me, "I lost my baby, and I lost my husband."

I had the distinct feeling she was clinically depressed, and felt sorry for her.

Ruth

Ruth, in the early/mid stage of the illness, is always in a good mood when I visit. Sometimes we get to laughing about something and end up laughing ourselves silly.

Ruth enjoys watching the birds at the bird feeder outside her window, which we often do together. She also likes to do crossword puzzles and is quite good at them.

Most of all, she enjoys playing with my Shih Tzu puppy, Christina, and I have taken Christina more than once. Ruth doesn't remember my name and doesn't remember that I visit every Thursday, but she remembers my puppy and frequently asks me to bring her in!

Ruth's husband is deceased, and she has three children. One lives in town and visits her frequently. The others visit when they are here.

She is very talented at making up rhyming lines to poems we write together. She also has a penchant for telling funny stories.

She once told me, "You're the only person around here I can have an intelligent conversation with!"

Among her dementia symptoms is her frequent mention of 'downstairs.' She thinks the facility has a downstairs but, in fact, it's all on one level.

She also often tells me, "Mary [her daughter] is coming from out of town to visit me soon."

This is despite the fact that Mary was just there and won't be returning for a few months.

We both regret it when it's time for me to leave. We have several parting rituals, including a big hug.

Daisy

Daisy's husband was still living at the time I visited her, and she had two daughters. Like Ruth, she tended to be in a good mood all the time. She dressed elegantly; she came from a well-to-do family.

One of her Alzheimer's symptoms was that she always believed and told me, "I'm going home tomorrow."

Daisy has since passed away after a bad fall from which she never recovered.

Ethel

Ethel, in the mid stages of Alzheimer's, was, above all, a talker! She seemed lonely, and she just loved doing 'show and tell.'

The minute I entered Ethel's room she would begin showing me the clothes she had made for herself, the quilt she'd made, and all of the pictures on her walls. This was accompanied by long descriptions of each item. Ethel was often quite confused but remembered details of her belongings.

She would tell me, "My family owns this facility." She would also tell me repeatedly, "My daughter will be home from school soon" and "I'm going to go to work in a bit."

One of her most endearing features was that she always called me 'Honey.'

She also said, "You're like a friend I can talk to. I sure do enjoy your visits, Honey."

One day after I left she stayed at her door and shouted, "Love you!" I answered back in kind.

Ethel later moved to another facility. I couldn't imagine why anyone would leave such a wonderful facility, and I miss the 'show and tell.'

Sue

Sue is painfully shy and tends to be rather serious. Never married, Sue has a good friend named Priscilla who takes care of her affairs and visits frequently.

Sue often tells me, "Priscilla is in charge of me."

Sue was a brilliant artist before she developed Alzheimer's, and many of her splendid works are on display in her room. They are breathtaking.

She often tells me, "I am no longer interested in drawing."

Her main activity is doing crossword puzzles. As is the case with Ruth, she is very good at them. Sue is extremely well educated.

Currently in the early stage of the disease, she displays no particularly distinguishing signs. I typically feel frustrated when I leave because I haven't yet found a good way to communicate with her or reach her on a significant level. I will keep trying.

Ann

Ann was in the late stage of Alzheimer's when I met her. Like Daisy, she'd suffered a fall, and as is often the case, never recovered. She had several children, but only one—a son—visited her. Unfortunately, he was a person she despised. I'd been told she was a very talented artist, but she had stopped painting by the time I met her.

This beautiful lady passed away after my fifth visit to her.

Maria

Maria, one of the recent additions to my visit list, is in the mid stages of the disease. She's very religious. She tells me she says the rosary and prays twice a day.

She loves to help people and always looks for an opportunity to do so. A social person, Maria spends most of her time in the common areas, participating in virtually every single activity.

Like Sue, she never married and has no children. She does have a few living relatives and is visited every week by her cousin.

Still, she tells me at every visit, "No one ever visits me." She always adds, however, "My family would visit if they thought I really needed anything."

Maria enjoys listening to Elvis. I take an Elvis CD with me every week and play it for her. It perks her right up. She loves it. After visiting Maria, I am always in a good mood, I think partly due to her pleasant nature and partly thanks to the lively music we listen to.

So these are 'My Ladies.' They have enriched my life immeasurably. I hope I've helped them, as well.

Chapter 11: Meet Daniel's Dad
Laying Down Roots

My father, Lester Eugene Potts, Jr., was born on November 4, 1928 in a logging camp in Camden, Mississippi.

Sawmilling was in his blood. It was a genetic memory. His ancestors had come to Itawamba County, Mississippi in the early 1800s to a saw milling settlement. The family eventually settled in Pickens County, Alabama in the 1890s, and Dad lived all but the last years of his life within 20 miles of the old home place.

It was in this sawmilling environment that my father was raised and learned the values of hard work, ethics, trust, and tolerance.

My father was a utilitarian child of the Great Depression. He valued his work ethic more than any other attribute, and labored as hard as he could all his life. He loved and trusted the men beside whom he toiled in the saw mill, and remained life-long friends and brothers with them. This brotherhood later deeply influenced me when, as a child, I witnessed the love and mutual respect displayed between two old friends—one black and one white—who reached deeply within and found kinship: Lester Potts and Albert Corder.

Dad claimed to have been strapped up like a mule and made to skid logs out of the woods as a young man. (Somehow, I doubted this claim!) He always seemed happy and at home in the woods, with a sapling stick in hand for protection, looking up at limbs that had always provided his shade.

I know very little about day-to-day life in Dad's childhood, except that there was work, family time, frugality, church, and good cooking. Dad's mother, 'Katie B.,' was apparently a good cook and homemaker. Though she died before I was born, I have heard she and Dad had a close bond and that she depended on and was proud of her son, Lester. In fact, it seems the whole family had a lot of faith, trust, and pride in Lester. He lived as if he was aware of this.

He never talked with me much about his childhood, but I got the feeling there was little leisure time. He mentioned sawmilling more than anything else. How hard the work was and how every man depended on the others to do his job. If each did not, injuries could result. Apparently, Dad had a close call one day when a board flew off the saw and hit him in the shoulder. This could have killed him.

Dad always talked about how tough and strong his father was and how he could outwork anyone at the mill. 'Big Daddy' (as we called Dad's father, Lester, Sr.) was the boss of the mill. 'Big Daddy' apparently used to pull a crosscut saw with Lester, and the old man would wear Dad out on the saw.

Some farming also took place, and cotton and corn was grown. I think there might have been some sorghum, too, and perhaps other crops. Dad talked about plowing with a mule, stopping by a spring for water, and picking cotton until dark.

Every time the doors were opened at Pine Grove Methodist Church, the Potts family was there. Dad actually led the singing for some time, a fact that is almost unbelievable to those of us who had heard him try to sing (though our opinions changed late in his life). There were lots of 'singings' and 'dinners-on-the-grounds' at Pine Grove, and the Methodist and Baptist churches were right across the road from each other, all shaded by the gnarly oak limbs of antiquity.

Church was the meeting ground for neighbors, as well. Apparently, Sunday afternoon visits were common on the community's porches. I sat on some of the same porches as a boy, rocking in some of the same swings.

Dad was a good basketball player, and he was captain of the varsity team when he was in high school. His complete ambidexterity had its advantages, both on the court and in the saw mill.

The earliest rings in Dad's oaken core were laid as he lived and worked and loved in this place. Times were hard, but I think they were also good. Themes from these early days were to emerge in poetic poignancy in Dad's late-stage watercolor art. I believe these themes and images helped to set the table of home for him later when he was slipping away due to Alzheimer's disease.

Growing a White Oak

Dad continued to work in the saw mill in the daytime and went to college at Mississippi State University at night. He graduated with a B.A. in business, the first person in his family to complete a college degree. He then partnered with his father in the saw mill. He left home for a couple of years to serve in the United States Army during the Korean War from 1950-52.

After basic training, he became a member of the Army's Corps of Engineers and was tasked with building missile silos in Alaska that were aimed across the Bering Strait at Russia. He drove an 18-wheeler loaded with these missiles from the mainland to the Alaskan coast. He often spoke of this, especially of the cold so uncommon to a boy from Alabama, and of the anxiety-producing treks through the Rocky Mountains loaded with missiles.

He returned home in 1952 and soon met the love of his life, my mother, Ethelda Oaks. They were married in 1959 in Columbus, Mississippi. My mother is a woman of culture: a musician, English teacher, and librarian. Though quite different in upbringing and gifts, their match was made well, and they spent almost 50 years together in love.

Starting out in Columbus, Mississippi, they moved to Aliceville, Alabama, 17 miles from where Dad was raised, and set up home there. Dad left the saw mill and bought an American Standard Oil dealership; Mother took a job teaching English. I was born from this union on January 27, 1966, and was to be my parents' only child.

Lester was the epitome of a solid citizen. He became one of the town's trusted leaders; everyone knew they could depend on 'old Les.' He was chairman of the Administrative Board at his Methodist church for 16 years, and Mother was the music director for 25.

He was each new minister's dear friend, and I always believed he would have welcomed the minister and his family to live in our home, if needed. He held claim to the left back pew at that church for 40 years, and was an usher most Sundays. He was a fixture at church clean up and repair days.

The Lions' Club was another of his passions, and he maintained perfect attendance nearly the entire time he lived in Aliceville. By virtue of Mother's extensive leadership activities and community involvement, Dad graciously assumed complementary roles as, for instance, the set-builder for the Aliceville Little Theatre (Mother was director), the piano mover for singing at church picnics (Mother was the church choir director), and the set-up guy for events at the library, where Mother served as librarian.

He was quite a handy fellow to have around. When anything quit working, he fixed it. I mean anything. We rarely had a repairman in the home. Lester never met a task he couldn't handle.

Watching Dad hammer a nail was poetry in motion. He could hammer with either hand, in any tight place, and if he bent the nail he could straighten it out with one side-armed strike of the hammer. It was amazing to watch him work. I held many a plank and steadied many a flashlight for him to do his magic.

Actually, he was always working, even when he was resting. There was rarely any idle time. And if he was expending energy, it was not in vain. He never understood the whole idea of setting aside a time for exercise, such as jogging. He thought this was a waste; one should be working up a sweat doing chores or helping someone else.

Lester also helped take care of folks. He didn't care what color your skin was, who your mama was, where you lived, whether or not you went to church, etc. He just loved people and considered them brothers or sisters. He treated everyone with respect and stood on level ground with all. His interactions were warm and loving, light-hearted and humorous, and uplifting. You couldn't leave a visit with Lester without a smile on your face. And his word was golden. Everyone knew that. They all wanted Lester on their team.

He was the kind of father I would have dreamed of having. He believed in me and was proud of me. He sacrificed in every way he could so that I could have a better life than most. He and Mother gave me every opportunity they could for growth. Dad never swayed or bent from what he felt was the right way.

Though we were in the ranks of the lower middle class, Dad knew almost every poor person in that part of the country. And they admired him because they knew he cared and was ready to help in any way he could.

Leaving the sawmilling business in the 1960s, Dad had other occupations, including owning and operating a service station, working at a cattle feed company, and managing a John Deere farm equipment dealership. His last job prior to retirement was as manager of a hardwood dry kiln operation for a large lumber company. When he retired, three men were hired to do his job.

My parents saved and sacrificed to send me to a private liberal arts college. With their unfailing support and encouragement, I chose to pursue a career in medicine and became a neurologist after completing residency training in 1997.

Dad's last act of citizenship and service in the town of Aliceville was to serve on the city council, which he was honored to do. With Lester at city hall, the citizens of his district knew they had an advocate of unquestioned integrity looking after their interests.

You see, Lester had grown into his favorite tree, the strong and useful Alabama white oak. And I grew into a man under its shade. I wouldn't trade anything for my childhood in that family, in that place, under that shade.

The Blight Sets in

After retiring, Dad took a job delivering newspapers to small towns in the region. I later found out from Mother that he had difficulty finding his way a time or two. Around this time, he found out the church trustees had voted to cut down a large magnolia tree in the churchyard. This angered him, and he proceeded to lambast them for cutting down the tree. This was quite uncharacteristic of him. We knew this at the time, but just chalked it up to caring a little too much about the tree.

Mother and Dad moved away from Aliceville in 2000 to be closer to me and my family in Tuscaloosa. Almost immediately, Dad got a job parking cars at a local office building. He also had minor surgery about that time and became delirious afterwards.

Unbeknownst to us, Dad was beginning to have trouble on the job. He started losing keys, locking keys in cars, losing cars, and getting lost in the parking deck so that his co-workers would have to look for him. He also had a few minor car accidents while traveling home.

Mother began to tell me she thought something might be wrong. I explained away this behavior, thinking it was due to the recent move, getting older, and having had anesthesia. But the behaviors got worse and were associated with short-term memory loss, confusion about time, difficulty managing finances, problems using his hands, and trouble expressing himself.

I received a call one day from Dad's employer asking to speak with me about his performance. In my office she told me what was going on at work and how they would have to let Dad go for his inability to perform his duties. She informed me that employment laws would have prevented her from coming to tell me these things, but that she felt this information was vital to share.

Pangs of reality then set in. Even though I was a neurologist, I had missed the opportunity to diagnose my Dad's disease and get him help as early as possible. I thanked her profusely, and prepared to enter a new phase of life— that of an Alzheimer's caregiver.

Dad called later that day and told me he wouldn't be working there anymore, that he had decided to just enjoy retirement with Mother. He hung up, and I cried. And I hung up, and he cried. For the very first time in my awareness, Lester was failing. He had let his co-workers down. He couldn't do what was asked of him. The blight had begun, and the day was dark.

Shoring up the Oak

A neurologist friend then gave Dad a diagnosis of Alzheimer's disease and started medication. Dad's course of illness was unusually rapid. He lost much of his language function early on and had to resort to 'pat' answers when responding to a greeting. For instance, if he was asked how he was doing, he might respond, after some hesitation, "I'm strong." Then he might flex a bicep to prove the point.

And strong he was, indeed. I once saw the man deadlift 200 pounds off the floor and press it, military-style, over his head— and that at age 70! The pronouncement, "I'm strong! I can put 200 pounds over my head. 200 pounds!" continued to be one of the few phrases he could easily think of to say (with accompanying hand motions, of course). Another was "I'm proud of you." I think this came from his nature as an encourager. Who knows? Maybe he was also seeking validation from those he met.

Dad progressively lost the use of his hands. Due to a phenomenon known as apraxia—the inability to perform learned tasks—he could no longer put lights on the Christmas tree or use a screwdriver to make repairs.

I think he could perceive what was happening to some extent, and this made him depressed. Mother would hear him crying as they knelt to pray. When she asked him why he was crying, he would say, "I'm so messed up."

He was rapidly losing his independence. In one year, he went from being able to recognize all but two road signs on a driving evaluation to being able to correctly identify only two. I'm sure he was tragically losing pride in himself and becoming ashamed. He stopped smiling and became depressed and apathetic.

In addition, he was becoming difficult for Mother to handle. He was big, strong, and physical, and if she got in his way he would simply push her away. This happened a few times, as did the attempts to wander outside, get up at 2:00 AM and start cooking, rearrange the furniture, etc.

Mother, through a Herculean effort, kept him at home without help as long as she could before it got to be too much. I almost had to insist she get help and respite. She agreed, and this help came in the form of an adult dementia daycare facility called Caring Days.

Caring Days (The Mal and Charlotte Moore Center) is one of the finest facilities of its kind in the country, and the only day facility in Alabama to receive the 'Excellence in Care Dementia Program of Distinction' award from the Alzheimer's Foundation of America. It receives support from more than 20 churches and synagogues in the Tuscaloosa area and provides safe, secure, affirming, and stimulating services for those with dementia of any cause.

Dad agreed to attend thanks to a little trickery. We told him, "Those old folks need you to help them, and they need some repairs done to the place." He bought into it and started attending in around 2002. We weren't sure how he would do, and Mother was skeptical, but we took him there anyway.

Vicki (the center's executive director) and Dad immediately hit it off and eventually became surrogate father/daughter. They loved and enjoyed each other and had such fun! I remember telling Vicki that I wished she had known Dad the way he was before. "I don't," she chuckled. "I love the Lester I have come to know right now."

And love him she and the other staff and clients certainly did. He loved them, too. Apparently, Les was the life of the party. He gave bear hugs and told everyone how strong he was, letting them feel his muscles. Once after he had hugged Vicki numerous times and told her he could put 200 pounds over his head, Vicki said, "Is that so, Les? What about 210 pounds?"

"Yep, I can put you over my head," he replied.

Because of Dad's sometimes dangerously strong displays of affection and to keep from sustaining broken ribs or separated shoulders, Vicki developed a plan. As Lester came at her with those big arms, ready to deliver a hug, she threw kisses instead. Dad would catch a kiss and throw it back, and this became an acceptable replacement for the bone-bashing bear hugs.

It didn't take long for this kind of person-centered, validating care to have a positive effect on Dad. He started smiling again and seemed to enjoy going to Caring Days. In fact, any time someone asked him where he was going, where he had been, and what he wanted to do on any given day, the answer was, "Caring Days."

Then the miracle occurred, and Lester's world would never be the same.

The Colors of the Fall

The program of cognitive enrichment at Caring Days included the arts: music, crafts, drama, and storytelling, all coupled with reminiscence. These modalities have been shown to be of benefit to those with dementia and can help to promote dignity and a higher quality of life. Dad certainly seemed to enjoy participating in all of these. Then along came the artist.

George, a retired visual artist who worked primarily in watercolors, was well-known in the Gulf coast region for his renditions of lighthouses, pelicans and gulls, fishing scenes, boats and riggings, etc. His works hang in restaurants, condos, hotels, and other facilities in the area.

George had apparently known his share of hardship and had had some serious health issues. He actually had a near-death experience and felt as though he had been touched and saved by God. As he was awakening and coming to some sense of self-awareness, he became strongly convinced that he he'd been saved for a purpose: to share his artistic gifts with persons who have dementia.

George then signed up to participate in a community outreach program and connected with Vicki, who had been looking for someone to start a visual arts program. George was not a trained art therapist, but possessed an uncanny natural inclination of how such therapy should occur, and so he started a watercolor program at Caring Days.

As far as I knew, my dad had no talent for painting. He also was no great appreciator of art. As I have often said, Dad was the fastest person though an art museum you have ever seen. He would be outside complaining about how expensive the gift shop merchandise was while Mother and I were reading every plaque and following every brushstroke in a gallery!

So the teacher met the pupil. Lester, a person with mid-stage Alzheimer's who could no longer hammer a nail, operate a screwdriver, lay out his own clothes, or complete a sentence, met George, a retired artist who had been shipwrecked in heaven, gotten directions from God, and was on a new mission. Beautiful treasures lay just ahead.

George started by getting the clients accustomed to watercolors, brushes, and other supplies. Then he put up images for them to copy, such as flowers and boats. He helped them draw the material in pencil and then choose paints. When he felt they were getting comfortable, he started letting them paint on their own. Then Lester's spirit began to soar.

Lester brought home his first completely original watercolor one afternoon around 2003. It was a picture of a hummingbird. Mother will tell you that she doubted he had painted it.

But he had.

Something very important happened that day that changed Lester's life for the better, instilled hope, and provided a wellspring of water for his roots. A new talent had been discovered, one that likely would have never been revealed without his Alzheimer's disease with its accompanying disinhibitions. Lester previously would have never let himself sit down and pick up a brush. It was aesthetic. Recreational.

Over the next few years, Lester painted more than one hundred original watercolors. He painted things that he remembered— images from childhood, from home. Familiar items and imagined ones. Things that had always brought joy and comfort and ones we had never seen.

When he was in the middle stages of Alzheimer's, he painted with amazing technical skill. This was made all the more unbelievable considering his advanced loss of visuospatial skills and dexterity. Something about the art freed his expression. It harnessed and honed his physical capabilities. He used the brightest and warmest of colors. Eventually, his art became more abstract and he tended to use only one or two colors in later stage works, usually green and blue.

Looking at Dad's late-stage art is like taking a tour through his life, especially the early years. At a time when his condition was so advanced that he could not craft any meaningful verbal expression, he was opening his inner sanctum to us through art.

The most poignant of all his works came near the end, just before he had to stop going to Caring Days because of progressive functional loss. In one of his depictions, two men are seen pulling a cross cut saw. One of the men is obviously Dad, a white man with a cap and white hair. The other is a black man who bears an uncanny resemblance to his life-long friend, Albert. When I saw the picture, I asked Dad if he was pulling the saw with Albert. He simply cried. Lester and Albert, in life and in art, were pulling the old saw together again.

The family's favorite watercolor is called 'The Blue Collage,' created when Dad was nearly bereft of language. Its depth and richness tell the story of his life, in abstract. In it one sees a house or a birdhouse, a fence, rocks, and leaves, etc. In the upper right-hand corner of the image, however, is a rendering a great importance, both artistically and spiritually.

Lester's father, 'Big Daddy,' was an easily recognizable figure. He always wore a hat and high-topped, lace-up shoes. He was also fundamentally a saw miller, a Christian, and had, of course, passed on many years before.

An abstract image of 'Big Daddy' appears in the upper right corner of the painting. 'Big Daddy' is wearing his high-topped shoes. A cross is coming out of his shoes, and a hat and a saw are coming out of the boot. Even more incredibly, the depiction was in the proportions that would appear to a small child crawling around on the floor. The high tops were big and the hat very small, as if seen from a distance.

Lester had crawled around and found his daddy again. He, like all persons with Alzheimer's disease, had been looking for home. And he had found it in the watercolors.

Dad continued to paint for a while after 'The Blue Collage' was created, but the pictures progressively lost color and form. He used certain perseverated themes in many of these later works. For instance, he tended to repeat a wood grain theme, as if looking at a log on end that had been sawed in two. This image certainly would have been laid down indelibly in his memory during his early life.

The art helped him access the memories that were still there, even though he could not create new memories.

Then, for the last rendering, devoid of any color, he drew a cross cut saw without the handles. It seems he strained out one last remnant of reality, a self-portrait of sorts— an object of steely tenacity and strong tensile strength, with handles worn off from labor and selfless giving.

The saw. He had painted a portrait of himself. As far as we know, he never painted anything of form after this, though he did continue to use watercolors for some time.

I never was able to see George and Dad interacting, though I know they had a deep relationship. The fruit of this is the art itself, revealed in all its depth and vibrant color. I think George and Dad were sailing on the same boat together, following homeward winds that wafted ceaselessly all their days.

As George came through the family receiving line after Dad's memorial service, I thanked him for sharing his art with my dad and for befriending him at a time when it was so hard to communicate with him.

By this time, Dad already was well-known in the Tuscaloosa area for his art. With a gleam in his eye, George responded "It was my pleasure and honor. And I will tell you, son, you haven't seen anything yet!"

Within the next month, George was dead. I never got to ask him what he meant by that comment, but I think I am beginning to find out.

Then Came the Winter

Soon after painting 'The Crosscut Saw,' Dad had to stop attending Caring Days due to his advancing condition. Looking back on it, his condition appeared to stabilize for about one and a half years while he attended Caring Days. I think this was due to the art and other person-centered care techniques he received there.

After his departure, his behavior worsened and he became a threat to himself and others. Dad had advanced past the point of being able to live at home, and we placed him in a series of assisted living facilities. He remained vigorous and physically strong, as well as modest. In short, he did not want to be 'messed with' during private times, and he lashed out, sending nurses and CNAs to the Emergency Department.

Only it wasn't him. Lester wouldn't do that. He would take you somewhere if you needed to go, and sit with you, and see about you, and tend to your family while you were there. It wasn't fair. It just wasn't him. But the staff didn't know that.

We knew what we had to do. We called our family friend, the Probate Judge of Pickens County, whose father-in-law had been the previous judge and a close friend. I later learned that the elder judge had said, "This one is special. It must be done with care and with the utmost respect. This is Lester Potts."

And it was done right. Commitment proceedings ensued in the Pickens County Courthouse with some of our attorney friends assisting. My former nurse practitioner, who had taken care of Dad, testified that he was a danger to himself and others.

Lester Potts a danger? To anyone? Damn this disease. Damn it straight to hell, I say.

Thanks to another friend and colleague who is a geriatric psychiatrist, we were able to secure a bed for acute stabilization at a geriatric psychiatric hospital, and there a peace ensued that would more or less be with Lester until the end. Those capable professionals did what they had to do to calm him, and he never was a threat to any of his caregivers again.

After about a month, we transitioned Lester to the Tuscaloosa Veterans Affairs dementia residential facility, and there he stayed until near the end. This was a caring, compassionate place with well-trained staff, and Dad spent those weeks in relative peace.

Caring Days' yearly fundraiser is the Walk to Remember, held every August at a local mall. Dad loved to attend this event. He could out-walk everyone. It also gave him the opportunity to hug many new unsuspecting subjects and to tell them he was strong.

But he got agitated in the crowd a couple of years before, so we had to stop taking him. Then in 2007, a month before Dad died,

Mother told me she would like to take him to the walk. I told her I did not feel this was a good idea, but she said she thought it might be the last time. So I agreed.

The wheelchair van pulled up outside the mall, and Lester was rolled in, wrapped up in a prayer blanket knitted by the women of First Presbyterian Church. By this time, his hands were contracted and he was nonverbal.

As he rolled through the mall, people began to stir and wanted to come over and speak to the local celebrity. He shook hands but made no other response. Vicki, who had not seen Dad in months, noticed him coming in, relinquished her duties as emcee, and headed through the crowd to greet old Les.

When she got near, she reached out and took his face with her hands, looked right into his eyes, and said "Lester Potts, I love you." That moment transcended time as they stared deeply into each other's eyes. Though Dad could not utter a word, Vicki communicated with him on a deep level. I think I heard the soul song. I will never forget that moment. That is what finding joy in a relationship is all about.

After we left the walk, we took Dad to my office, where prints of his art were hanging. He had never been to my office to see them. We parked him in front of one of his favorites that we call 'The Broken Jar.' Amazingly, he stayed there for thirty minutes staring at the work. He never said a word, but I certainly hope he recognized it on some level, and that he reconnected with a part of himself that was expressed in the painting.

Dad's hidden artistic gift brought many benefits. It made his depression decrease, helped calm his agitation, improved his ability to perform activities of daily living, and helped make him be more alert and communicative. I think it temporarily helped stabilize his cognition, as well. It enabled Dad to express things at a time when he was losing his language skills.

The overall and most important benefit was that it seemed to improve his quality of life, shore up his sense of self, and restore pride and dignity to a broken man. It also gave respite to my mother as it helped his functioning, behavior, mood, and cognition, making him easier to care for. Furthermore, it fostered communication and interaction between Mother and Dad, which provided the added benefit of improving her quality of life.

Beyond the Sunset

During his last weekend at the VA facility, while I was giving Mother some respite, I had the opportunity to sit with Dad, look him in the eye, and tell him everything I had wanted to say, hoping he would understand on a deep level just how much he meant to me.

This was a privilege for which I will be thankful for the rest of my life. "You're the most wonderful man I've ever known. I hope I can be half the father to my girls that you are to me. You are a righteous oak. We will always love you. You don't have to hold on for us. Don't cry, Papa. It's okay. It's all right."

The death grip tightened, and aspiration pneumonia sent him to the hospital for the last of many times in September 2007. It soon became apparent that the end was nearing, and his attending physician approached Mother about the possibility of engaging hospice care.

I cannot begin to imagine the agony a spouse of nearly 50 years must experience when trying to make such a decision. But she did, and I am proud of her. She had kept him at home long past the time it was reasonable for her to do so. She stayed by his side until the end. She fed his body and soul with mighty good things.

As he moved to Hospice of West Alabama's Helen H. Hahn House, I went down to prepare the room while Mother stayed with Dad. From the moment of entry, the warmth of this place wraps one up like a quilt from home. The halls are lined with the most beautiful paintings, all from local artists, which help create a feeling of warmth and beauty.

The staff and volunteers there are cut from that same cloth. I am not able to praise them enough. Angels they were, every one. And they came to Mother and comforted her about letting go. About loosening her grip so that he could clasp the hand of Another.

Seeking to create an air of familiarity, I placed prints of Dad's paintings and old family pictures on easels around the room so that everywhere he looked he would catch a glimpse of something he knew: the sunset picture, 'The Broken Jar,' 'The Blue Collage,' and many of his other paintings. I also placed his high school graduation picture, a photo of his mom and dad, and pictures of his loving bride so that he could see them. I wanted him to see them. To feel their eyes and arms reaching out to him. I just wanted him to feel at home.

For the next four days, Dad's room was a holy place of song, prayer, and anointing. His bed remained encircled by family and friends and those who had cared about him. The old fellow was showered with as much pure good as we could round up for him, because we all knew he deserved every bit of it and more.

Mama fed him well. We told him what we thought of him, and it was all as good as he was. He was alert and responsive to us, though non-verbal. The preachers came. He always loved his preachers. We sang every hymn he knew, and he sang with us. Yes, he sang. Despite the fact that he couldn't talk, he sang.

About mid-afternoon on Friday, September 14th, things changed. He spiked a fever, and his difficult breathing worsened. He began to look more distant and somewhat anxious. By late that afternoon, I suspected this would be his last full day on earth. During this time, he began to focus upward toward the corner where the ceiling and the wall met, but just short of that point to the surrounding air.

After he had sustained a fixed gaze on that spot for over an hour, I asked the family and friends what they thought he was looking at. I decided to ask him, expecting no response from this man who had not been able to utter a sentence in weeks.

"Papa, what are you looking at?" I said.

Then he turned his head and eyes toward me, looked me straight on, and uttered, "Mama."

He then turned his face back to the ethereal spot. We bowed down in our hearts at the timeless mystery of that moment and of the manifold comforts in death.

A short while later, sensing the hour of death approaching, Mother and I hunkered in for a night of woe and triumph. Everyone left, and we were all alone, the three of us, just like in the old days.

Death by aspiration pneumonia is not for the faint of heart. He was so strong and held to life so tightly. That made it tougher. I've seen death many times up close. I've been there for the struggles, the gut-wrenching, blood-stilling rattles, and the heart-shocking, chest-crashing struggle of it. But it's different when it happens to flesh of your flesh. It just is.

Several times we cried, "How long, O Lord? How long?"

God was with us. I saw His eyes. Everything was bowing down to pure love, and God was in that room with us.

At last, at 4:15 AM on September 15th, 2007, the beautiful soul of Lester Eugene Potts, Jr., a saw miller and watercolor artist, departed this world and entered into the eternal light of God.

Since Dad's death, his story has inspired me to create of a foundation, Cognitive Dynamics, whose mission is to improve the quality of life of persons with cognitive disorders (such as Alzheimer's disease) and their caregivers through education, research, and support of innovative care models that promote human dignity, especially therapies employing the expressive arts and storytelling.

Through this foundation we are now bringing art therapy to community-dwelling persons with Alzheimer's disease, preserving the life stories of these individuals to enhance their quality of life, and promoting the growth of empathy in my college students for those with dementia and their caregivers.

Lester Potts' art has been shown internationally, and his story of hope amidst suffering continues to inspire, bring joy, and demonstrate that personhood persists despite the affliction of Alzheimer's disease.

Chapter 12: Stories of Love and Acceptance

<u>The Finest Part</u>

> In the very thought of you, toil itself found rest,
>
> saving what it caught of you for some later test.
>
> Visions that would calm the mind, still the stirring heart:
>
> tranquil faces, ever kind; love, the finest part.
>
> Daniel

The 'Lee-tle' Yellow One

(Marie)

I knew I'd never be able to accept Ed's Alzheimer's. It was so bad I couldn't have a meaningful two-way exchange with him. He couldn't advise me about my problems or praise me for my successes as he'd always done. He couldn't provide emotional support and be that solid rock who had always been there for me.

One morning before going to the nursing home to visit him, I stopped by Walgreen's to buy some shampoo. To get the shampoo, I had to pass the stuffed animal section. I had no idea why, but those sweet little playthings caught my eye and brought Ed to mind.

Would he like a stuffed animal? I asked myself. He was childlike at times.

I immediately told myself I was crazy, and that he'd feel insulted and become irate if I gave him a stuffed animal. Finally, on a whim and against my better judgment, I decided to buy him one. I chose a miniature yellow chick. When you pressed a little red button on its chest it said, "Peep, peep, peep."

On the way to the nursing home, I kept wondering what an elderly man was going to do with a stuffed animal that peeped. That former erudite scholar, lawyer, and professor of French. The man who'd had such a brilliant mind.

I arrived and greeted Ed.

"I brought you a present today, Ed," I said.

I held the chick for him to see, then handed it to him. I didn't have to wait long for his reaction. His eyes began to sparkle, and a look of wonder came to his face.

I showed him how to push the little red button. He started laughing and pushing the button repeatedly, putting the chick to his ear each time.

"Mar-r-rie, I can't thank you enough," he said. "You help me so much, and now you brought me this wonderful present."

"I think you should give it a name," I said.

"The 'Lee-tle' Yellow One!" he announced with glee.

"I'm coming to visit you again tomorrow," I said, changing the subject.

"Oh, I'm delighted!" he said. And then he asked, "Do you know who else is delighted?"

"No. Who?"

"The 'Lee-tle' Yellow One!"

It was clear he was aware and proud he'd said something amusing.

Hearing the excitement in his voice, I decided to take a chance and asked, "Would you like a bunny rabbit, too?"

"Oh, yes! I would love a bunny r-r-rabbit because he would be a companion for the 'Lee-tle' Yellow One."

So I decided that if stuffed animals gave him so much pleasure maybe I'd keep bringing him other, similar presents. It wasn't the kind of interaction with him I'd been wanting all those months, but I guessed it would be better than sitting in silence, feeling dejected and unloved during my visits.

On my way home, I realized that when I'd experienced his joy at that tiny stuffed animal my heart began to be transformed. Gradually, my need and desire for my 'old Ed' began melting away as I realized that I could bring such happiness to my 'new Ed.' The man who had lost so much was in a state of child-like bliss thanks to my small gift.

I eventually became aware that little by little and without noticing, I had accepted his illness, and I had found new ways to relate to him, ways that were genuinely satisfying for both of us. Just seeing him smile and hearing him laugh had become more than enough to make up for losing our previous relationship. My heart had changed forever. Our love had adapted and endured, despite that last and most daunting obstacle it would ever face.

I Love You

(Marie)

It is often said that animals and children reach people with dementia on a deep level.

Every time Ed saw my little Shih Tzu, Peter, he said, "Oh, the 'Lee-tle' one. I love him so much."

I often took Peter with me to the Alois Center where Ed was living. Most of the time, as soon as we'd enter the lobby, Peter was the center of attention. Tom would suddenly smile, which made me smile, too. Carol would cradle her teddy bear in her left arm, lean down, and pet Peter with her right hand. I knew Joyce liked Peter, but since her eyesight was so poor, she couldn't see him, so I'd pick him up and hold him close to her face.

One day I arrived and found Ed dozing in his wheelchair, as had become usual by that time.

"Hi, Ed. Here we are," I said, certain my voice was loud enough to awaken him.

He lifted his head and looked at us.

"Oh, the 'Lee-tle' one," he said, emphasizing 'Lee-tle,' and perking right up. "'Pe-tair. Lee-tle Pe-tair'. Come here," he said, reaching out his arms. "Let me see you."

Ed didn't even look at me.

"'Lee-tle' one. 'Pe-tair,' come here," he repeated.

Peter ran to Ed.

"Hi, Marie," he said, finally turning his attention to me. "Can I hold 'Pe-tair?'"

"Sure."

I put 'Lee-tle Pe-tair' on Ed's lap as I had done so many times before.

Mary, the housekeeper, came in, wearing a lovely sunflower blue pullover and navy slacks. She emptied the waste basket.

"Hi, Peter," she said in the tone of voice people often use when talking to a child.

Almost all the staff knew Peter by name.

"Looks like you've got a good buddy there, Edward," Mary laughed. "I bet he'd like to move in here with you."

Ed laughed, too. His laugh sounded artificial. That was how I knew he hadn't understood what she'd said and only laughed because she had.

"I have to go on to the next room now, Ed."

"When are you coming back?" he asked.

"Soon," she promised.

"Wonderful!"

After Mary left, Peter put his chin back on Ed's arm, and Ed resumed stroking him.

"Does he like it when I 'pad' him?" Ed asked, looking at me expectantly.

"Yes, he likes to be petted."

"Oh, I'm so happy he's happy when I'm 'padding' him."

When it was time to leave, I started slowly putting on my jacket.

"I love you," Ed said quietly.

I was startled. We'd never said those words to each other. We knew it and never felt the need to say it.

"I love you, too," I said simply, looking in his eyes.

"When are you coming back?"

"Tomorrow," I answered as always, zipping up my jacket. I wasn't planning on coming back the next day, but I knew he'd never know the difference, and it made him happy.

"Marvelous! Wonderful!" he exclaimed.

Expecting a Gift
(Daniel)

It can't be all giving. We must be open to receiving, as well.

When my father started attending Caring Days, the adult dementia daycare center where he learned to paint, we were thankful that he was receiving the most compassionate and validating care possible, delivered in a joyful, enriching environment.

It was apparent that he needed this kind of care. He certainly received it and benefitted greatly, but we didn't expect him to be able to give back. He was the broken one who needed all the help, wasn't he?

After a few weeks, the positive change in Dad was clear. He smiled more, became more communicative, less anxious, and more engaged. He seemed to have pride in himself again.

We were so thankful to the staff at the center and expressed our gratitude to them. What we heard back from them was unexpected.

It seemed that the staff and clients at the center had received a gift from Dad, as well. It turns out he blessed them with his loving and encouraging nature, warmth, and good humor. They all looked forward to seeing old Les come in the front door each day. He brightened the place with his spirit. Why had we not expected that?

Then came the art. Although he had never painted before receiving his Alzheimer's diagnosis, Dad's artistic gift was expressed in more than a hundred watercolors that he painted during his time there. The one who needed help became the giver, and I became the recipient of that gift.

As I have alluded to previously, I struggled mightily with Dad's illness, with what I perceived as my failure to recognize the early signs, and with my inability to support Mother the way I felt I should. Wanting to help, I gave as much of my time, energy, and knowledge as I could, and still felt inadequate.

Paradoxically, I found myself on the receiving end of inspiration, comfort, and joy through Dad's art. It spoke to a very deep place in me and brought so much healing. It was this gift that kindled my desire to express myself through writing. In turn, I was energized and encouraged to be a better caregiver. All of this produced an unexpected joy that could then be infused into my relationship with Dad and our visits together.

"It is in giving that we receive," said St. Francis of Assisi, but as caregivers, we must be open to this receiving. We must expect a blessing in return. The truth is that if we only see ourselves on the giving end we likely will experience burn-out, and this will take away our joy.

This experience with my father taught me something profound that has continued to instruct me over the years and has become one of the primary themes I share when speaking with other caregivers. The inspiration and energy required to be our best as caregivers comes from the very ones for whom we are caring.

There is reciprocity in any healthy relationship. When we find ourselves in this state of giving and receiving, we find ourselves. This is also true for those who have Alzheimer's and other dementias. The loss of cognitive functions does not diminish their capacity for relationships. We owe it to our loved ones and to ourselves to believe this.

Healthy relationships built on this balance of giving and receiving produce inner joy, which infuses itself back into the relationship and spreads out to others.

Each time we come into the presence of someone who has Alzheimer's disease or another dementia, we should do so expecting a gift from them. This will make it much easier for us to have a joyful experience during our visits with them.

Two Men With Alzheimer's Connect

(Marie)

I remember reading somewhere that people who have Alzheimer's enjoy being with others who also have the condition. The following story clearly illustrates that.

When I went to visit one day, I found Ed in his room looking at the newspaper, which he was holding upside down.

When he saw me he exclaimed, "Oh, Marie, I'm so happy to see you. You are so beautiful." Then he added, "Since I became in such high admiration of you, other beauties didn't exist."

I was amazed that given his state of dementia he could still express himself so poetically.

He folded the newspaper carefully and placed it just so in the top desk drawer. Then he walked over and sat down on the Early American sofa the Alois Center had provided until I could get his furniture moved in.

I sat down beside him, crossed my legs, and propped my feet up on the coffee table. We discussed the horrible conditions in New Orleans, which he kept referring to as 'New Jersey,' after Katrina had hit just days before.

Suddenly, a stocky little man appeared in the doorway. His black trousers hung a couple of inches below his waist, and his plaid burgundy and grey flannel shirt was un-tucked on the right side.

I was surprised when Ed, a life-long loner, smiled and reached out his right arm then shouted, "Come in. Come in.'"

Ed looked at me and said, "Marie, this is my dear friend, John. We've been best friends for years."

John shuffled in, advancing in short jerky movements, his house-slippered feet barely lifting from the floor. Slightly balding, his remaining hair was jet black, his eyes dark brown, and he had a round jovial face that reminded me of my Irish Grandpa Graves.

"Yes, we've been best friends forever," John said, waving at us.

Ed patted the empty space next to him on the other side of the sofa and John sat down. Then—and you might imagine my shock—they started holding hands and taking turns telling me how many years they'd been best friends.

They reminded me of two little girls sitting on a bench, dangling their legs while waiting for the school bus. I was delighted—though dazed—that Ed had made a friend, and so quickly, at that. Ed had never been one to make friends at all. And he'd only been at the center a week. They sat there talking—small talk, actually—and they continued holding hands. It was something we rarely, if ever, see in today's society, but it seemed perfectly natural for them.

"Hi, John," I said, wanting to be gracious to Ed's new friend. "How long have you lived here at the Alois Center?"

He snapped to attention. "All my life," he answered proudly.

I shouldn't have been surprised, but for some reason I hadn't expected this man to be as confused as Ed.

After a while, John said he had to leave. After exchanging more pleasantries with Ed, he let go of Ed's hand and stood up. He bid goodbye to his dear friend, then exited in the same shuffling gait with which he'd entered.

The whole incident made me feel warm inside, and I knew then that I'd done the right thing by moving Ed to the Alois Center. It was obvious that he needed and enjoyed the company of other people.

I peered out the door and watched as John inched down the hall and disappeared into another room, which I assumed was his.

I found myself hoping he'd come back on a regular basis to visit Ed, his dear, affectionate 'childhood friend.'

The Innate Human Capacity to Feel Joy (Marie)

I went to visit Ed one Sunday. It turned out to be a special, joyous visit. I wish I were a great writer and could fully describe the essence of the visit, but I am not, so I will just do the best I can.

After a pleasant drive to the Alois Center on that crisp fall day, I arrived and walked down the hall to Ed's room, wondering what type of mood he was in that day.

When he first saw me his eyes lit up and he said, "Oh, it's you! Oh, I am so happy to see you! You are an angel! I am overwhelmed to see you! Oh, I am overwhelmed!"

He moved with his walker from his rocking chair to the Early American sofa and patted the empty space beside him, indicating that I should sit there, so I did.

He took my hand and kissed it several times, continuing to say he was overwhelmed and didn't have words to say how happy he was to see me.

His eyes were shining, his face was full of joy, and he held my hand, kissing it again from time to time. That was so typical of Ed, ever the quintessential European gentleman.

He was so happy that he was near tears. I don't have words to describe how his joy and his being near tears at the same time combined to make a powerful and joyful experience for me.

While we were still sitting on the sofa, I picked up the 'Lee-tle' Yellow One, his most beloved stuffed animal, and handed it to him. He reacted joyfully and as though he had never seen it before.

"Oh, the 'Lee-tle' one. I love him so much!" (He referred to all of his stuffed animals as 'him.')

His eyes lit up again and he petted the little animal with loving strokes and then kissed it several times on the top of the head with an affectionate expression on his face.

His extreme joy to see me and his intense love for the little stuffed animal affected me to my core. I was so happy to see Ed in that wonderful state of being, and I felt warm inside all the way home.

If only we all could feel such joy from a simple visit from a friend.

"I Like That Kind!"
(Daniel)

The need for relationships is our deepest need.

Spiritual and faith traditions teach that the desire for a relationship with God, a 'Higher Power,' Being, or Consciousness (terms for essentially the same Entity) is the primary longing that underlies our quest for the fullness of life. This need extends to our relationships with humans, other living beings, and even the inanimate world around us.

Relationships help us define our core identity, revealing to us and to the universe who we are.

This deep need for relationships does not go away when people develop Alzheimer's disease or another dementia. In fact, it actually becomes more pressing as the disease begins to cut one's ties to others, and even to oneself, through attacking memory and other elements of cognition.

Those of us who have loved someone throughout the perilous march of dementia have experienced the challenges of maintaining meaningful relationships late into the course of the disease. Though challenging, it is still possible. And not only possible, it can be rewarding and a source of growth for caregivers.

For relationships to be maintained, we must believe people with Alzheimer's still retain their personhood. They are 'still there,' though it may seem otherwise at times.

They are stamped with an incontrovertible identity and innate dignity that nothing can take away. If we don't espouse that view, then it will be hard to engage them in a relationship.

Additionally, for relationships to work we have to look for the essential elements of their personhood. What makes them who they are? What are their likes and dislikes? What characteristics define them and shape the way they interact with the world? What are their most important values, and how have they expressed them in their lives? What matters most to them? What are their talents and gifts? What, and whom, do they love?

My wife, Ellen, is no novice when it comes to experiencing dementia in family members. As a young girl she witnessed Alzheimer's creep into the life and mind of her maternal grandfather in the days before the disease was well understood. This made a profound impact on her and brings home the importance of multigenerational efforts to educate and support caregivers of all ages.

Ellen's paternal grandmother, Margaret ('Maggie' to close relations), was a pillar of her community in northeastern Tennessee. A homemaker, teacher, and church leader with deep family roots in the history of that region, she moved from her beloved Appalachia after the death of her husband to be near her son (Ellen's father) and his family in Huntsville, Alabama.

From all I have heard Ellen and other family members say about Maggie, she was a dear, sweet soul and a Southern Lady to the core. Graceful, kind, humble, and a great cook, she was deeply loved in her community. It didn't take long for her strength of character and her love and integrity to endear her to a growing circle of friends in her new home.

But Maggie began to experience that startlingly subtle but steadily advancing loss of cognitive function that marks the path of

Alzheimer's. Showing rare insight and humility, she voluntarily gave up her car keys and made the decision to move into a residential care facility. What a gift that was to those who cared for her!

I was only fortunate enough to know Maggie during the last few years of her life when she was confined to bed or a reclining wheelchair. She rarely spoke and sometimes was not fully aware or alert when we visited.

But I was able to know Maggie through the loving way her granddaughter, Ellen, engaged her in a relationship.

When we entered the room, Ellen would move toward her grandmother in a way that demonstrated full presence of being: gentle, compassionate, and joyful, expecting Maggie's spirit to reach out in a loving embrace like she did when Ellen would run to greet her as a little girl.

"Hey, Grandmama! How are you today? We're here to see you. We're so glad to see you today!"

Ellen touched her lovingly, spoke softly and sweetly, paying full attention to Maggie and looking into her eyes at eye level. She told her what was going on in her life and the lives of those who meant a lot to her. Grandparents want to know about the lives of their grandchildren, and Maggie looked at Ellen, listened, and occasionally smiled.

Those smiles were a gift that Ellen will hold onto. And so will I.

Ellen sang to Maggie, fed her, prayed with her, and expressed love to her in any way she could. It all was tailored to what she knew of the essential personal traits of her grandmother, and it didn't matter that Maggie didn't say much anymore. Words mainly express thoughts, but being there and being present expresses much more.

The first time I got to meet Maggie was right before Ellen and I married, and Ellen wanted to tell Maggie of our upcoming wedding and introduce Maggie to the new fiancé. What an honor for me to meet this lady I had heard so much about!

After her usual methods of engaging Maggie in the moment, Ellen asked me to come closer to the bedside. Knowing that her grandmother had been a life-long Methodist until she moved to Alabama and joined the Presbyterian Church where her son and his family attended (a big surprise to her family!), Ellen chose to introduce me while tapping into that trait that helped to define Maggie's identity.

"Grandmama, I want you to meet my fiancé, Danny. He and I will be getting married soon. And Grandmama, I think you will really like him. He is a good Methodist boy!"

Old Maggie brightened, straightened up in her bed, got a big smile on her face, and beamed at the strange young man standing at her bedside who would soon receive her granddaughter's hand in marriage.

"Oh, I like that kind!" she surprised us all by saying.

From that point on, I had a meaningful relationship with this woman who was very much still with us, was very much in need of relationships and love, and was very much capable of extending the warmth of her spirit to those who took the time and made the effort to be present for her in the 'now' of her existence.

You see, the 'now' of her existence had nothing to do with Alzheimer's disease and everything to do with who Maggie still was.

I like that kind of 'now.'

I hope to remember what Maggie and her granddaughter, Ellen, have taught me as I seek relationships with other Maggies I will meet along the way.

A Special Relationship
(Marie)

I had just returned home from my weekly visits with My 'Ladies', and was sitting lost in thought. Lost in the memory of my just-completed visit to Ruth. I know I shouldn't have a favorite, but I do. Ruth is my favorite.

She was quite confused that day. She told me that she had tried to rent an apartment that she liked very much, but before she could conclude the deal they 'fixed it up' for someone else. I knew that wasn't true, but I empathized with her. "Oh, I'm so sorry," I said.

Then I changed the subject to something pleasant. "I see you have some See's candy here. Do you want a piece?"

"Oh, yes," she said. "Will you have a piece with me?"

"Of course," I answered. "Gimme that box!"

After eating more pieces than I can say without embarrassing myself, I told her to save me some for next week. She promised she would, and we laughed as we hid the box so no one else would come in and eat 'my' candy.

We then discussed a wide range of topics. She told me her son had locked her car in the garage so she couldn't drive any more. Again I empathized with her, and again I subsequently changed the conversation to something more pleasant. We went right back and started laughing and talking about that candy and where we'd hidden it.

When I finally told her it was time for me to leave, she got a pouty look on her face and asked, "Oh, do you have to go?"

"Yes, I'm afraid I have to leave now. I wish I didn't, but I'll come back and see you next week."

"What day?" she asked me.

"Thursday," I said.

"Thursday. I'll try to remember that."

"Oh," I said, "You don't have to remember. I'll find you." Then I added jokingly, "I'll hunt you down and find you wherever you are!"

We both laughed, and she seemed relieved she wouldn't have to remember what day I was coming back.

Then she walked with me to the door. She put her arms around me and hugged me tightly.

"Oh, I sure am glad you stopped by. I depend on you. You're my friend," she said.

"I love coming to see you," I said.

Then I stood back and looked at her. Her eyes were brimming with tears. I was touched and hugged her again. Then we went through our usual parting ritual and she cheered up.

"See you later," I said.

"Alligator," she said, a twinkle in her eyes.

"After while," I continued.

Without missing a beat she jumped in and said, "Crocodile."

"See you next week," I told her as I went out the door.

"See you," she said, smiling and gently closing her door.

This is why I volunteer. I felt warm all the way home, and I was looking forward to the next week when I could 'find' the candy and enjoy some. But mostly I was looking forward to seeing Ruth again and experiencing the warmth, love, and joy we have in our special relationship.

The Art of Listening
(Daniel)

"The deepest level of communication is not communication, but communion. It is wordless—My dear, we are already one."

Thomas Merton

In medical school and during residency training we were taught the importance of listening. Granted, by observing some of the master clinicians who were my teachers, I came to understand what good listening skills were like, but honing them myself was a different matter altogether. That skill developed primarily from my relationships with people who have Alzheimer's.

The disease affects one's ability to communicate with words. Not only can words become more difficult to think of and produce in speech, but also word meanings may be lost, causing all sorts of communication problems.

In some cases of dementia, this loss of semantics, or word meaning, may make it difficult for a person to understand and express the emotional content of words. At one time or another, most of us have had trouble recalling someone's name. This phenomenon, as well as difficulty naming objects or parts of objects, quite commonly shows up as a symptom of Alzheimer's disease.

The problems just described come under the term aphasia, which is the inability to understand or express language. This is one of the core characteristics of Alzheimer's disease, and it renders communication challenging, at best.

But we communicate in ways other than through language, don't we? In fact, at times non-verbal communication may be more expressive or truthful than verbal. This form of communication becomes especially important in persons with Alzheimer's disease and other dementias, and in those of us who seek meaningful, joy-filled relationships with them.

We have to learn to develop the skill of non-verbal communication and to become good listeners.

I teach a course called 'Art to Life' at the University of Alabama Honors College. In this course (inspired by my father's story and artistic gift), students are paired with persons who have Alzheimer's disease in an art therapy experience. Students learn about the disease, about art and other expressive therapies and their benefits, and about person-centered caregiving and the importance of life stories in the delivery of such care.

During the semester, students learn and document the life stories of their participants. More importantly, they develop empathy for people with Alzheimer's disease and build relationships with them.

Recently, the students and I got to practice good listening techniques, and in doing so we received a great gift.

John, a participant in his early 70s with moderately advanced Alzheimer's disease, has fairly prominent expressive aphasia. There are long pauses when he is trying to share his thoughts.

At first, I could detect some frustration and discomfort in the students, who weren't sure what to do when he was struggling for words. After the first art therapy session, we talked about this and discussed our strategy for handling it during the next session.

I shared with them what I had been told by several people with Alzheimer's disease over the years: they did not want to be interrupted and helped to complete their sentences if they were searching for words. Instead, they wanted to be given time to come up with the words themselves, and they expressed their frustration at being denied the opportunity to actually say what they meant, despite the good intentions of the 'helpers.'

In a subsequent session, we were able to practice our skills. The art activity in which John was participating reminded him of an experience he wanted to share. As he started telling us about it, he was having a hard time coming up with the words. There were long pauses during which we all had an urge to supply words for him.

But it seemed these pauses were only awkward to us. John did not look frustrated. He continued telling his story at his own pace. The students and I had talked about mindful listening: engaging actively and non-judgmentally in the moment and the content contained therein, being completely present in mind, body, and spirit, and listening for anything that was being communicated verbally or nonverbally.

So we waited for him to speak, being careful not to express anxiety or impatience in our facial expressions or other body language while maintaining intense attention to what he was telling us with his whole person. And this soon paid off.

The further John got into his story, the better he was able to verbally express himself. The students and I could see this clearly, and it was a beautiful thing to experience.

When John finished telling us his story (which happened to be about an important event in his life in which he had been able to offer assistance to others in need), he had a look of satisfaction and joy on his face. He seemed proud of himself, and we were proud of him, too.

In our later discussions about this, we realized that our mindful listening practice had given John the space and encouragement he needed to express himself, and he had been validated as a person in the process. What he had to say was important enough to wait for.

This kind of listening had required us to step out of ourselves and into his world, and we had been enriched by the experience.

Learning to be good listeners will increase our capacity to experience joy and to share it as we develop relationships with people who have Alzheimer's.

The Poetic Voice of Alzheimer's

(Daniel)

I met Cathie Borrie shortly after my father passed away from Alzheimer's disease. As many do, I reached out to other caregivers in my passion to make a difference in the cause of Alzheimer's and dementia advocacy.

What I had heard of Cathie's story deeply resonated with me. We soon were able to meet in person when I traveled to Vancouver in 2012 to interview her for a planned documentary on finding the people inside the disease and building a relationship with them. I discovered that Cathie knows more about that than almost anyone else.

In her profoundly stirring memoir, *The Long Hello*, Cathie shares the heart and life of her mother, Jo, as she newly discovered her through her caregiving. An intelligent, strong, and artistically gifted lover of fishing and birds, Jo survived her first marriage to an alcoholic husband and the death of her young son. Later in her life, Jo was diagnosed with Alzheimer's and Parkinson's disease.

Through many missteps in her attempt to bring back the voice of the mother she had always known, Cathie learned to 'listen a different way.' As Jo's condition progressed, Jo began to express herself more and more in poignant poetic lines, freshly revealing the still vibrant life force dancing within her. This gave Cathie a new avenue through which to relate to her mother.

Writing the first few words of her 'mum's' new language on coffee-stained serviettes, Cathie began recording their conversations, and a story soon took shape.

"I am choreographing a dance for my mother and me," Cathie told her therapist.

Deftly crafting her mother's ethereal lines with her own wandering feelings and tender triumphs, Cathie weaves a story so rich that it fills the canvas of caregiving with dark and deep colors like the bird-speckled Pacific waters she and her mother sat gazing across for long periods of time.

Cathie: "What are the birds saying?"

Jo: "They're chirping."

Cathie: "In a language?"

Jo: "In their language. In an upside-down language."

Though Cathie finds respite in her mother's new voice, pain still pierces Cathie's gut. Courageous yet vulnerable, Cathie shares the naked hurt pounding inside while she tries to lose herself in a ballroom dance class.

"Let me ask you, what do you think is the ugliest thing in the world?" Cathie asks her mum.

"A lack of dignity. Is that the right answer?" These words of Jo's make me think of my father.

Though dark and deep, Jo's days are laced with humor that is so refreshing to those of us who have walked this road.

"You're my favorite person in the world," chimes Cathie.

"Favorite amongst the constipated, you mean…" retorts Jo.

Facing a health crisis of her own (so common among caregivers), Cathie calls out from beneath the weight of complete responsibility for the well-being of another person, feeling alone and inadequate to perform the task. Using the metaphor of dance, she explains:

"Men complain that women try to lead and that's why we go the wrong way on the dance floor, why feet get stepped on. I go the wrong way because I'm afraid of doing something stupid or because I miss the lead signals. I don't know how to do nothing. Be empty enough, quiet enough inside to wait. To listen. I can't believe someone else will take care of the leading. Take care of anything."

In absorbing this beautiful memoir, one can clearly appreciate that Cathie did, indeed, succeed in choreographing a dance for the two of them. In doing so, Cathie gave her mum the freedom to speak in her real voice despite dementia's onslaught. One must know when to lead and when to follow.

As this story reveals itself page by page, we see that the true lead belongs to Jo, the very one being crippled by dementia, yet whose spirit is emergent even amidst faltering steps. Cathie lets the spirit do its dancing, and then lets her own join in joyful relationship.

"It's always easier to remember the lines when you understand the story," Cathie says. Cathie understands the story—her mum's, her own, and ours.

Love Remembered Despite Alzheimer's (Marie)

I wandered into Ed's room one day and found he was in his bathroom, so I sat in the rocker and waited.

That day I'd decided to show Ed the cards and photos I'd found in his storage unit while I was cleaning it out. It was my friend Rosa's idea. I never would have thought of doing that myself.

"Ma-r-r-rie!" he exclaimed, coming out of the bathroom. "I'm r-r-really happy to see you. You are so beautiful!"

Then he sat down, careful not to disturb the little stuffed animals on the sofa.

"Ed, I found some old photos and cards that I sent you many years ago, and I'm going to show them to you today."

"Marvelous! Superb!" he answered, using the words he always used when he was happy about something.

I decided to start with the cards. Although he was no longer able to read books or the newspaper, I hoped he'd still be capable of reading the cards. He was, and he even seemed to understand what he read. He laughed at the funny ones and responded more seriously to the others.

After he'd seen them all he looked up at me and said in a reverent tone of voice, "Ma-r-r-rie, I am so touched that you kept these cards all these years."

I didn't even try explaining that he was the one who had kept them.

Next we looked at the photographs. Some were from his childhood. There was one of him around age six wearing a sailor suit and posing with his father, and another with him and his grandparents sitting on a bench in a beautiful park.

Then there were several pictures of Ed with me from the '80s and '90s. There were also photos of him with a whole variety of people I didn't know. I guessed they were different Romanian friends and relatives.

He was drawn to the photos just as much as he was to the cards, studying each with interest.

The last one was a picture of him from 1985 with a woman standing behind him. She had her hands on his shoulders and her head was peeking around his, facing the camera.

"Ah… She loved me," he murmured, an affectionate expression on his face. He appeared mesmerized and kept looking at the photo in silence.

I was stunned. He didn't realize that I was the woman in the photo, but he remembered vividly that the woman in the picture had loved him. He remembered and experienced the affect.

"What are you thinking?" I asked when he didn't say anything more.

"I'm thinking of love," he said softly.

"I'm that woman, and I still love you."

He looked up and gazed into my eyes exactly the way he did when we were intimately involved all those many years earlier.

I couldn't tell if he was in the past or the present.

I decided it didn't matter.

Lessons Learned From
Stories About Love, Affection, and Acceptance

1. When you accept the fact that a loved one has Alzheimer's, you may begin to have joyous visits with him.

2. People who have Alzheimer's may be able to remember, experience, and express love.

3. People with Alzheimer's tend to lose their sense of inhibition and may engage in lovely behaviors they never before would have. (Unfortunately, they may also engage in challenging behaviors they wouldn't have before.)

4. Those who have Alzheimer's may enjoy spending time with others who have the disease.

5. Placement in an assisted living or long-term care facility offers many opportunities for socialization that may not be available at home.

6. Those with Alzheimer's may still have the capacity to feel joy.

7. People with Alzheimer's may enjoy activities they didn't like before developing the illness. (Conversely, they may not enjoy things they did like before.)

8. Simple activities may bring happiness both to the loved one and the caregiver.

9. People who have Alzheimer's may be quite alert, even if they don't talk anymore.

10. You may have to experiment to find a way to reach a loved one with Alzheimer's.

11. If you listen, you will receive messages from your loved one who has Alzheimer's, even in the later stages.

12. Expect to receive blessings in your relationships with people who have Alzheimer's.

Chapter 13: Humorous Stories

<u>We're Here!</u>

In my tear

you saw reflections of yourself

that made you laugh.

Then I started grinning.

"Horton Hears a Who!" you said,

and sparkled like a little one heard.

We chuckled together 'til nightfall,

having found the hidden cache.

     Daniel

Laughing with Lola

(Daniel)

Everyone in town called her 'Aunt Lola,' but no one knew whose aunt she really was. She was simply ours.

Dad said Aunt Lola had always been an interesting bird. Of course, things got a bit more interesting later in her life when Lola began to develop Alzheimer's.

Aunt Lola lived in a rural area, and her husband, Uncle Buddy, had passed away a few years before. She eventually transitioned into residential care, but for a few years she lived by herself in her home, within a few miles of other family members who checked on her and who kept us entertained with Aunt Lola stories.

If I seem to approach this in a lighthearted manner, it's because that's the way Aunt Lola would want me to. As concerned as we all were about her delusional thinking, memory loss, and confusion, these issues did not bother her at all, and she spent most of her time laughing and cheering up everyone else.

She experienced several paranoid delusions, and the content of them was the topic of most of the conversations in which Aunt Lola engaged herself.

"They came and got my Irish potatoes and brought them back cooked!"

"Someone has been in the refrigerator and fingered my chicken salad sandwiches."

"I came around the corner and there he was—a man in a strange suit."

As she related these tales of home intrusions and clandestine food operations, she did not appear to be overly concerned, was redirected easily, and usually would gravitate toward some topic she thought was funny.

In a minute or two, we were all laughing with her, sometimes to the point of tears.

Aunt Lola never took herself or her problems so seriously that she couldn't share a little cheer with friends and loved ones. When Aunt Lola laughed, you had to follow suit.

Soon the laughter took on a life of its own, and you were no longer sure exactly what you had been laughing about.

In reality, it would have been difficult to have anything but joyful visits with Aunt Lola. All we needed to do was follow her lead and engage ourselves to go where she headed.

We need not be afraid of the concept of play. Play is necessary for all of us, even as we age. It is an activity and mindset that is centered in the present and requires a detachment from fear, judgment, and goal-directed planning to enjoy each moment in carefree gaiety. I enjoyed playing with Aunt Lola!

The delusions died down as her disease advanced, and Aunt Lola eventually had to be placed in a residential care facility. However, she was still full of joy and laughter, even as the curtain of Alzheimer's progressively decreased her understanding. She still laughed and she still smiled, and she did so more heartily when others chimed in with her.

Toward the end, I could tell she was getting weaker, and some of that spirit with which we had been so familiar started to be silenced a bit. Laughter came, though not as vivaciously, but her innate trait of seeking relationships, of reaching out from inside herself to clasp the hand of another never faded.

Laughter and joy are always more meaningful when shared. Aunt Lola knew this in a very deep place, and from that place, she continued to laugh and experience joy until the very end.

Aunt Lola taught me the importance of laughter and play in our lives, even as we age, and that I should never take myself and my personal issues too seriously.

A Brief Walk on the Light Side of Dementia (Marie)

I'm going to share two amusing stories about Ed. He also found them funny, and we both had a good laugh!

An Alzheimer's Sneaky Thief

After finishing each meal at the Alois Center, Ed would always carefully wipe his spoon clean with a napkin then wrap the spoon in another napkin, put it in the breast pocket of his sport coat, and take it back to his room.

Pretty soon, his room would have spoons all over the place, so the staff would go get them and return them to the kitchen. But sure enough, the next day he would start a new collection.

Finally, one day when he started his cleaning ritual I said to him, "Don't take that spoon, Ed. It doesn't belong to you. It belongs to the Alois Center."

"Oh, no!" he said, loudly enough for everyone to hear. "I take them every day with no remorse!"

He was aware he'd said something funny, and we burst into laughter.

The Little Pillows

Spoons weren't the only thing Ed pilfered. They had sofas in the lobby that had little designer pillows on them. For some reason, Ed was drawn to those little pillows (or 'pee-lows' as he pronounced it) and developed the habit of taking them back to his room.

Just as with the spoons, the staff would go to his room periodically, retrieve all the little pillows, and return them to the sofas. And just as with the spoons, he would begin stealing them all over the very next day.

One day I was sitting with him in the dining room when one of the kitchen staff members, Ann, came over to say hello to us.

I said to Ed, "You really enjoy stealing your spoons, don't you?"

"Yes, he certainly does," said Ann.

Just then Ed got a sly grin on his face.

"It isn't just the spoons I steal," he said proudly in his thick Romanian accent. "I also r-r-really love to take those 'lee-tle pee-lows'!"

He began laughing and so did Ann and I, and you guessed it, he kept right on stealing the spoons and the 'pee-lows'!

Bring Me Vodka!

(Marie)

One day I went to visit Ed. When it was time for his dinner I left, walking him to the dining room on my way out.

"Marie, please bring me two bottles of Popov tomorrow," Ed said sweetly as we passed the dining room.

Ed had always enjoyed drinking, and vodka was his preferred drink.

"Ed, I can't," I said, my body stiffening in anticipation of the ugly scene I knew would follow. "You're not allowed to have vodka here."

"What do you mean, I'm not allowed to have vodka?" he asked incredulously.

He stopped walking and glared at me.

"This is America! I'm allowed to have anything I want!"

"I'm sorry, Ed," I said, my voice wavering. "I can't bring you any. That's the rule here."

"I don't need you!" he shouted. "I will find someone else to get it for me. And you can be sure I will r-r-remember this!"

I winced. I didn't want a major scene, and I knew I couldn't win the battle so, as much as it hurt, I turned my back on him and rushed out. I felt embarrassed as I passed Alice, the aide who was setting the tables.

I felt hurt when I went out to my car. As I drove home, I felt sorry for Ed. I knew how much he needed his vodka, and I wondered if he'd ever adjust to not having it.

A few hours later Ed called me and, as though nothing had happened between us, cheerfully asked me the address of "this place where I am 'leev-ing.'"

Digging in my wallet to find the social worker's card, I was pleased. I thought it was a good sign that he wanted to be oriented and know where he was. I told him the address, and he repeated it one letter and number at a time, leading me to think he was writing it down, which I also thought was a good thing.

The minute I hung up I got it.

Oh, no! He's going to call Mr. Ellington, his 'driver,' to take him to buy some vodka.

I dialed Ellington's cell phone as fast as my fingers would move and explained the situation. Mr. Ellington promised to tell Ed his cab had broken down and it would take him a few days to get there. Mr. Ellington was a dear.

I must admit, however, I was pleased Ed was still alert enough to figure out how to try to get some vodka. I checked with Ellington later and found out that Ed had indeed called him.

A few days later, I met briefly with Michelle, the director of nursing.

"By the way, Michelle, you'll never guess what Ed did the other night," I began. "He tricked me into giving him this address, and then he called a cab to take him to buy some vodka! Fortunately, I had the cab driver's cell phone number, so I called and told him not to come. I don't know what would have happened if I hadn't had his number."

"Oh, Marie," she said, leaning against her office doorway, laughing. "Don't ever worry about anything like that. We'd never let Ed go out without calling you first."

Then I burst into laughter, too.

Enough!

(Marie)

"Bingo!" a woman hollered in a shrill voice.

I peeked into the activity room and saw Ed smiling. He was sitting on the far side of the long craft table and looked like he was having a grand time. I didn't want to interfere with his fun, so I pulled up a chair and sat down beside him, planning to just observe. Martha, a tiny, sweet-looking aide, spun the cage, picked up the ball, and called out the combination.

"B-6!"

Ed looked at his card intently then sang out sweetly, "Here 'tis!" and covered the proper square with a red plastic marker. Quite frankly, I was surprised, but pleased, he was able to play without assistance.

Martha had seated Lucy and Sylvia on either side of her, so she could lean over and help them look for the numbers on their cards. Betty, at least ninety and almost as underweight as Ed, sat undisturbed amid the players.

The game continued, and each time Ed had the number he called out melodically with glee, "Here 'tis."

I found this amusing and had to suppress a laugh. Martha seemed to find it funny, too, and looked in Ed's direction, a smile on her face every time he voiced his little refrain.

Sylvia yelled something, in what I would later find out was Portuguese, in a disgruntled tone of voice every time she didn't have the required letter and number. I could tell Ed was getting annoyed with her.

Finally, I guess he decided he'd had enough of her grouchiness, because he said so loudly that it was embarrassing, "I have one word to say!"

"What is it, Ed?" Martha inquired, a concerned look on her face.

He pointed his shaky finger at Sylvia and shouted, "Enough!"

He was right. He did have just one word to say. It was clear he was aware he'd said something amusing. We all laughed with Ed, not at him.

People Who Have Alzheimer's May Say the Darnedest Things
(Marie)

My experience is that people living with Alzheimer's can say some pretty amusing things. Many times the person is aware and even proud that he has said something humorous. These moments can be among the most precious we will ever have with our loved ones. Here are some examples.

My first stories are about Ruth. Ruth tells me the same stories every time I visit her, except she sometimes includes new information or adds a twist to some part of them.

During one visit, she told me that during World War II the Army used to 'bus' young ladies to a base overseas on Friday nights to dance with the soldiers. (Of course they weren't sent overseas, but I didn't tell her that.)

"I was one of those girls. I must say that I was a great dancer, unlike many of the men," she said. "Most of them couldn't dance well," she continued, "and they just 'stomped out' a two-step."

When she told me that, she imitated the men in a most humorous way, merrily stomping her feet up and down.

Ruth also told me, "When we girls arrived at the base, the men looked us up and down like they were shopping."

That made us both laugh out loud.

One of the bits of information she added during a subsequent visit was, "My husband was an especially bad dancer. So bad," she said, "I think he must have learned how to dance in a barn."

As I was leaving one of my visits to Ruth, I said, "See you later."

She cracked me up when she said, "Alligator."

So now every time I leave we go through that little routine, even though sometimes I have to prompt her.

Then there was Ethel. My dear sweet, talkative Ethel. One day when I was visiting her, she looked at me curiously and announced, "I think you're my age."

And that despite the fact that I'm 20 years younger. I told one of the staff members about it. She was initially mortified, but then we both had a good laugh about it.

A final example of humorous things people with Alzheimer's said is involves one of my friends' grandfather, George.

It seems George was having a lot of trouble driving.

"I'll never stop driving," he always said adamantly.

And so my friend, Sandra, disabled George's car. George was, however, still alert enough to call a mechanic to come and repair it.

Sandra had assumed he'd do that, so she had called his mechanic the day before.

"Please give Grandpa some excuse for not being able to fix the car," she requested.

When George contacted the mechanic the next day, the mechanic told George, "Your car needs some parts that are only available on the internet. It will take a long time."

George then called his granddaughter and said, "Sandra, I have a job for you. Drive me to the internet!"

The Spelling Bee
(Daniel)

Transitions in dementia care can be very tough. Moving your loved one from home to a long-term care setting, or from residential care to a hospital, or to acute care and back again can be stressful for all involved.

Persons with dementia like stability, familiarity, and routine and need to feel they have some mastery over their environments. So this uprooting can set them back for a time, adversely affecting their behavior, mood, and mental clarity.

During these transitions it becomes especially important to employ any tools you have to lessen the stress. One such tool is role playing.

In your interactions with your loved ones, it is important that you be willing to enter their worlds, which will often be very different from yours.

For instance, loved ones may feel they are living in an earlier time, and they may believe that relatives or friends who have passed on are alive and in a relationship with them in the present.

Naomi Feil, the founder of Validation Therapy, teaches that this may be due to unmet needs.

"I want to see my mother," you may hear your loved one say. Perhaps he needs to be in a relationship with his mother and to be comforted by a familiar person who knows and understands him; who loves him just as he is.

People with Alzheimer's should be allowed to express their needs and to be in care environments that enable them to have their needs met in a non-judgmental, safe, and supportive way.

Similarly, loved ones may imagine themselves to be in a particular situation or activity from their past. As long as it is safe to do so, and if it appears to be comforting to them, it is important that they be able to view themselves in this way.

We were able to make use of the tool of role playing during one of my father's transitions. Dad had been living at home with my mother and attending an adult dementia daycare center. However, due to our safety concerns and Dad's increased need for around-the-clock support, we had to move him to a specialty care assisted living facility (SCALF).

In accordance with the intake and admission procedures for this facility, Dad had to be interviewed by the staff. The Mini-Mental Status Examination (MMSE), with which some of you may be familiar, was administered as a part of this interview.

Dad had taken the exam several times before during his visits to other healthcare providers, but his response on that day and at that particular time in his journey through the condition, gave our family a subsequent opportunity to engage him via role playing.

Dad was asked the standard questions, such as, "What day is this? What month? What year? What is the name of this city? This state?" etc.

When asked the following question, Dad's response brought smiles to our faces and ushered us into our new roles in his world:

"Mr. Potts, spell WORLD, backwards."

Dad thought a moment then replied, "BACKWARDS. B-A-C-K-W-A-R-D-S…BACKWARDS."

A spelling bee! In his world, Dad was back in grammar school participating in a spelling bee, and he appeared to be quite good at it. This was particularly surprising, since he already had lost the ability to read and write.

Our daughters, who were elementary school-aged themselves, were the first to happily assume their roles.

"Papa, spell 'ALABAMA.' "

"ALABAMA. A-L-A-B-A-M-A. ALABAMA."

"That's great, Papa! My Papa is a good speller," bragged our younger daughter, beaming.

And now Papa was beaming, too.

Thus, we were given a new activity to carry out in subsequent visits to Papa in his new long-term care residence. Not only did this opportunity for role playing help to ease the transition that day, but it also gave us a joyous activity to which we could return for many weeks afterward. It seemed to be fun for Dad and rarely failed to engage him.

It also provided an opportunity to build upon the theme of reminiscence, which is one of the most important themes in dementia caregiving.

In addition, it revealed Dad's previously unknown talent for spelling at a time when he was losing many of his mental faculties. This affirmed him in his present state and gave him confidence.

Furthermore, it helped to maintain and strengthen his relationships, especially intergenerational ones, such as those with his grandchildren.

This is critical, as the perceived loss of relationships may be the most important of the many losses experienced by persons with dementia and their families. I feel it is essential that persons with dementia be given opportunities to be in relationships with children and young people, and this activity promoted that kind of relationship.

When navigating those inevitable transitions with your loved one, be open to opportunities to enter his world and role play. You may be surprised at the joy that can be shared through such activities.

Maria's New Walker
(Marie)

When I went to visit Maria one day, I found her in the 'Hearth Room,' as they call it. It's a sort of combined dining room/lounge area where many of Clare Bridge's social activities are held.

I should mention that Maria is a deeply religious lady who carries two rosaries with her at all times, says the rosary twice a day, and is forever doing little things around the place to help other residents and even the staff.

She was sitting at a table with two other ladies, both of whom were beautifully dressed and looked confused. Maria herself looked quite angry—a mood in which I'd never before seen her.

I sat down beside her and asked, "Is something wrong, Maria?"

"No," she said, sounding as angry as she looked.

I resigned myself to not knowing what had caused her bad mood, and I just sat there watching the two ladies eat the brownies they had been served as part of the 'Mix and Mingle.' That is a Thursday afternoon activity in which the residents sit at tables and have—or in some cases, attempt to have—polite conversation with each other while eating the marvelous snacks they are served.

At a certain moment, I noticed Maria had a walker parked in front of her. I'd never seen it before, and it had a note taped to it on a large piece of paper with extra-large handwriting.

I couldn't quite read it from where I was sitting, so I asked, "What's that big note say, Maria?"

She painstakingly read the note to me: "Maria must have this walker with her at all times."

Without missing a beat, this prim and proper lady looked up at me and pronounced loudly, "That's bull #%&$!"

To the Mortuary!

(Marie)

It was almost Christmas, and Clare Bridge was all abuzz with holiday music. Colorful wreaths were appended to the residents' doors, and a large, beautifully-decorated Christmas tree adorned the lobby.

I sauntered down to Ruth's room and entered as she opened her own wreathed door for me.

"Oh," she said, "It's you! Come in. How are you today?"

Ruth doesn't remember my name and doesn't remember that I visit every Thursday, but she always recognizes me and knows that I'm someone she enjoys seeing.

"I'm great," I answered. "How are you doing?"

"Oh, I'm fine, fine, fine," she said.

At her insistence, I sat down in her comfortable armchair while she perched on one of her armless dining room chairs across from me. She always insisted that I take her armchair, the best seat in the room. I'd long since given up trying to convince her otherwise.

We were chatting away and at a certain point she said, "I don't know how long I'm going to be here."

"Where are you going?" I asked, bewildered by her statement.

She paused an instant then blurted out, "To the mortuary!"

We both cracked up. I told her that wasn't true and she shouldn't talk like that.

Later on, I spontaneously told her, "I don't know how long I'm going to be here."

"Where on earth are you going?" she asked.

I immediately pronounced, "To the mortuary!" We both burst out laughing, then I pointed at her and said, "Gotcha!"

Without missing a beat, she said, "You'll be going there to say goodbye to me!"

We then laughed even harder than before. It was indeed a joyous visit.

What If You Had a Fire in Your Kitchen?

(Marie)

One day before Ed moved to the Alois Center, I was with him at his apartment. He answered a knock on his door and found a pretty young lady in her mid-20s standing there. He smiled and gestured for her to enter. "Hello there! Oh, I'm so excited to see you again. How have you been? Come in! Come in!" he told her.

Only thing was, Ed had never seen her before. That alone pretty much fulfilled the purpose of her visit. Kristi, director of admissions at the Alois Center, was there to evaluate Ed for placement.

I'd warned her I couldn't promise he'd even allow her in, let alone talk with her, so I was immensely relieved he was agreeable that day.

Ed was oblivious to the real reason I'd arranged this interview. I had told him she was a friend of mine who worked in a nursing home and she wanted to practice interviewing elderly people. This was just another of the white lies I had to tell him to get what I wanted and he needed. It was only because of his dementia that I had to do it, and it was only because of his dementia that I could get away with it.

He sat in his recliner, which served as the centerpiece of the living room, and from which he watched his precious political talk shows.

Kristi, whose white summer dress was flecked with little green flowers matching the freshness of the sunny and breezy late

August day, took a seat on the sofa near Ed's chair. Not wanting to interfere, I sat at the far end of the sofa, planning to just observe.

Kristi explained the real reason she was there. Ed didn't seem to understand, but he was in an excellent mood and readily agreed to talk with her. I assumed it was mostly because she was so young and pretty. He loved all young and pretty girls.

Kristi consulted the paper that was attached to a manila folder with a large paper clip, turned her body directly toward Ed, and began asking the usual questions, enunciating each word clearly and loudly.

"Can you tell me who the President is?"

"Boosh," he blurted out, grinning.

"Can you tell me what the date is today?"

He thought for a few seconds, then his head began to slowly shift downward as he simultaneously turned his left wrist inward a little.

Well, I'd be darned! His mind isn't totally gone. He's alert enough to remember his Timex has the date on it.

That gave me some comfort. He stated the correct date, and we all three laughed about his cleverness.

"What state are we in?" she continued.

He appeared confused and looked at me.

"Sorry, Ed," I said. You have to answer by yourself."

"I'm so sorry," he said, looking back toward Kristi. "I really can't remember. I think it may be Ohio. Or Cleveland."

"Okay," she said. "What country do we live in?"

"America!" he shouted with glee.

"That's right! Now, can you count backwards by sevens, starting at 100?"

He had a blank look on his face.

"Count how?"

"Backwards."

"I can count very well—in English, Romanian, French, German, Russian, and Italian."

"Can you count backwards in English by sevens, starting at 100?" she repeated.

He looked at me again.

"I'm sorry, but I can't help you, Ed."

"I don't understand the question," he told Kristi, sounding flustered.

"That's okay," she said. "Let's go on to the next question."

"Certainly!"

"Can you spell the word 'world' backwards?"

He thought a moment then answered, "w – o – r – l - d."

"That's spelling it forward, Ed. Can you spell it backwards—starting with the last letter?"

"Well," he answered, "the last letter is 'I'."

I hoped I wasn't looking disappointed.

She continued with her questions and wrote down everything he said.

"Ma-r-rie is such a good and dear old friend of mine," he told Kristi after one of her questions.

"I think Marie loves you very much," she said quietly.

Kristi then asked the last question: "What would you do if you had a fire in your kitchen?"

He thought for a minute, then a sly grin slowly appeared on his face. He stretched out his arm, pointed to me with his shaky finger, and proudly announced, "I'd call her."

It was obvious that he was perfectly well aware he'd said something humorous and again, we all three had a good laugh.

Lessons Learned From Humorous Visits

1. People with Alzheimer's may be humorous at times and often realize it.

2. We can laugh with people who have Alzheimer's—not at them.

3. Sometimes laughter is the best medicine for both the caregiver and the person with dementia.

4. People who have Alzheimer's may at times be very clever.

6. Finding humor in a stressful situation can help to redirect attention and behavior.

8. Humor can establish islands of respite and safety in the sea of Alzheimer's.

10. We shouldn't listen to the voice that tells us to feel guilty for laughing.

11. Moments of humor are to be remembered and cherished forever.

Chapter 14: Stories About Special Activities

To Live

> To live
> is to learn the soul song
> and sing it
> to the world.
>
> Daniel

Please Wear a Tux

(Marie)

"Please wear a tux," I said over the phone to Don, the classical violinist I was hiring to play a special concert for Ed in his room at the Alois Center. As we were talking, I described Ed's state of dementia, adding that he had been a college professor of French who loved classical 'moo-sic.'

When I arrived at Ed's room the day of the concert, I was relieved to see the aide had shaved him and dressed him nicely in a light blue shirt and his grey tweed sport coat, the one with leather patches on the elbows.

After a few minutes, Don appeared in the doorway. I introduced Don and told Ed he was going to play a special violin concert for him.

"Oh! Superb! Wonderful! I'm honored!" Ed said as he shook Don's hand.

I had the feeling Ed was really impressed by the tux.

I set up my tripod. I planned to take many pictures, hoping to get at least a few good shots of what I hoped was going to be a special occasion.

Don sat down on the tan metal folding chair I'd placed in front of Ed and began playing a Strauss waltz. The sounds were lively and luscious. I watched as his bow flew up and down and his fingers danced around. Ed looked captivated. His eyes glued to Don, he had a rapt expression on his face and moved in time with the music.

"Bravo! Bravo!" he boomed in his bass voice while clapping at the end of the waltz. "That was the most beautiful 'moo-sic' I have ever heard in my entire, r-r-really long, and I emphasize r-r-really long, life."

Don thanked him and began playing a Romanian piece, as I'd requested. Ed smiled broadly, but I couldn't tell if he realized it was music from his homeland.

"Bravo! Bravo!" he called out again, clapping as before. "That was the most beautiful 'moo-sic' I've heard," he said. "Ever," he added. "I don't have words to say how happy I am that you are playing just for me."

"Thanks," Don said. "I'm glad you liked it."

Ed reached his hand toward Don, and Don grasped and held it.

"What did you teach when you were a professor?" Don asked.

"I don't r-r-remember," Ed answered. Then he added, "Honestly, I'm not even sure I was a professor."

Then, since there were so many Gypsies in Romania and that was part of Ed's culture, I asked Don to play some Gypsy music. He played Bizet's Habañera from *Carmen*, and Ed sang along, jabbing his index finger in the air in time with the music.

"Tra la la-la, la la la la-la," he sang, a twinkle in his eyes.

"Bravo! Bravo!" he shouted at the end of the piece. "That was the most beautiful 'moo-sic' I have ever heard in my entire r-r-really long, and I emphasize r-r-really long, life," he said again. "You are the most talented 'moo-si-cian' ever, and I r-r-really mean it from my heart. It's not just words from my lips."

Don played half an hour longer, the music interspersed with more hand holding and small talk. When the concert was finished, I asked Don to sit on the sofa beside Ed so I could take a picture of them. Ed put his hand on Don's arm, and I snapped the photo.

Don left after many more goodbyes, more excited compliments from Ed, and thanks from me.

Some of the photographs are adorable. Ed looked as happy as I'd ever seen him. One of the pictures shows him with both arms outstretched toward Don as he was playing. Another, taken when they were sitting on the sofa, shows Ed with his hand on Don's arm, looking as proud as if he were sitting next to the President or the Queen of England.

The pictures captured the happiness of a man who had lost so much, yet was still capable of great joy. He was a man who wouldn't remember the concert even an hour later, but he was captivated and delighted by every second of it as it happened, and that's what mattered.

I'm Proud of Your Art!
(Daniel)

It was my gold medal. My arrival in the winners' circle. My degree, with honors.

"I'm proud of you!" Dad beamed.

It didn't matter whether I had just gotten my first report card 'A,' hit a home run, sung my first solo, won a scholarship, or graduated from medical school. It always made me feel the same way: like I was sitting on top of the world, completely affirmed by my father's love.

And I wasn't the only recipient of his up-building words. Old Lester had a knack for knowing who needed a lift.

The main reason his praise meant so much was the integrity that we knew was behind it. He was as fine a human being as I will ever know. He could recognize what was good in others, and he told them he was proud of them. They were better people because he did.

After we had traveled with him a ways down the road of Alzheimer's disease, sometimes his affirming phrases became a source of embarrassment. I can remember several outings in which Dad approached total strangers, grabbed them, and told them he was proud of them. I wish I could have captured some of the perplexed facial expressions resulting from his proud pronouncements!

This phrase and a few others, like "I'm strong" became his pat responses and greetings after the diagnosis. I suppose he couldn't think of anything else to say. Perhaps, unconsciously, he wanted someone to say they were proud of him, too.

I got my chance the day he brought home the painting of the little hummingbird.

By the time we enrolled Dad as a client at Caring Days Adult Dementia Daycare Center, he had stopped smiling. He seemed depressed and defeated.

From his first days at Caring Days, Dad changed. He was validated in his current state by people who had no predetermined ideas about what he could or could not do. They saw a Lester of limitless possibilities. A strong man with boundless capacity for relationships. And they provided ample opportunity and an encouraging environment for those relationships to grow.

Dad soon met George, a retired Gulf Coast artist who started an art program for the clients. We had heard about the program, but we knew Dad wouldn't want to participate.

Then he brought home a 9" x 14" canvas on which appeared the most beautiful watercolor painting of a hummingbird with a bright red head, dark green wings, and a deep purple and yellow-striped body. It looked like a spiritual bird soaring up to the Heavenly realms.

"Look what I did," he said to Mother.

"Oh, Honey, who gave you that lovely little hummingbird? Did Mr. Parker paint that for you?"

"No, I did it. I painted it myself!"

The old man beamed like a little boy after his first homerun. He could do things he had never done before. He could paint, and he hadn't even known it!

All this was at a time when he couldn't use a screwdriver to fix the garden gate or place lights on the Christmas tree.

Oh no. Alzheimer's disease wouldn't be the end of Lester Potts! There was way too much wholeness left within him, although we certainly didn't recognize it at the time.

The old saw miller who had never painted a picture produced more than a hundred original watercolors during the next few years. Family and friends were amazed, and a man who thought he was broken had something for which to be proud again.

Though expressive language was leaving him, the art spoke volumes: his life story in vibrant hues, laden with images from his childhood. Birds, saws, woodgrain, his father's shoes, fences.

He painted home, he painted family, and he painted from that little boy's brain that still played inside.

He gained quite a following once his talent became known. Local art events served as a venue to show his work, and he was so honored. He loved to show those pieces to anyone who would pause, often time and again within just a few minutes!

Our younger daughter, just a few years old at the time, knew her 'papa' as an artist. Lester's friends from younger days, when they heard about 'Lester Potts the painter,' thought for sure a different person was being referred to. The old Lester Potts they knew could saw a log, not paint a canvas.

The art improved his condition. His depression and communication improved, and he was less agitated and more alert. He became easier to engage in a relationship, and this improved life for Mother and for the rest of us as well.

His art seemed to comfort and inspire those who viewed it. Our family has continued to hear story after story about how Dad's art spoke to people. Interestingly, it has seemed particularly effective in reaching people who have dementia. I wonder if they are seeing inside themselves some of the things he had seen and captured on canvas.

After Dad's death, his art and story began to take on a life of their own. At the time of this writing, they have been featured in medical textbooks, printed and digital collections of art, devotionals, catalogues and documentaries, and museums and conferences. They have appeared in venues from Beverly Hills to Paris. Thousands of people have been inspired by Dad's paintings, a foundation has been started, songs and poems have been written, and educational curricula have been developed around his artwork.

It all started with the little hummingbird he brought home, which at first we didn't believe he had actually painted.

When I saw it, I was greatly moved. He was still with us, after all. The beauty of that spirit I had known and loved—the same spirit that had drawn me close, lifted me up, and supported and protected me all of my life—now seemed to lift off the page and take flight.

He was leaving the disease and all of its problems behind. We seemed to take flight with him.

I was so very, very proud. Now, I could say so.

"Papa, I am so proud of you!" He knew I meant it.

I gave him back the gold he had given me so many times before.

And he wore it well.

'Conducting' a Visit

(Marie)

One day when I visited Ed I decided to play some classical music for him. After we talked a while, I put on a CD of the last movement of Mozart's *Jupiter Symphony*. Ed's eyes sparkled, his whole face beamed, he sat up straight, and moved in time with the music.

Then, for some reason I can't explain, I decided to pretend to be conducting the music. I was greatly surprised by his reaction. It made him smile broadly.

As I was 'conducting' with an imaginary baton, I recalled that years before he'd always enjoyed watching conductors on TV, especially the flamboyant ones. The wilder they were, the more he loved watching them.

As a musician, I knew that when conductors were showy, they didn't necessarily make the orchestra play any better, but I decided to emulate that type of conductor.

I conducted with both hands, arms flying around, sometimes in tandem, other times going in opposite directions. I pretended I had a baton in my right hand, cueing each section of the orchestra when it was time for their entrances.

Ed moved perfectly in time with the music, which impressed me. Typically those days he couldn't seem to do anything that well.

I stretched out both arms and bounced up and down when the music was loud, then crouched down and conducted in a tiny area, using only my right hand when the music was soft. When the music was at its softest, I put my left index finger up to my lips in a "shh" gesture while my right hand continued conducting in small circles. He laughed out loud at these motions.

After the final chord, I made a gigantic cut off movement, remained completely immobile for a few seconds, then bowed deeply—first to the right, then center, then left.

Ed, who had been sitting in the rocking chair during the entire theatrical production, looked positively radiant.

After my final bow, he looked at me and whispered in an almost reverent tone of voice, "What you did was so beautiful."

Many people had told me to listen to music with Ed, but I had always thought that would be boring. How wrong I'd been! Listening to Mozart with Ed was anything but boring. It had opened up a whole new way to relate to him and had brought him great joy, which made me feel joy, as well. I delighted in the knowledge that I had made him happy.

After this improvised concert, I became determined to relate to Ed in whatever way I could. I decided to continue these performances he loved so much. I later found out from the staff that he was in an unusually good mood for the rest of the day.

The Little Stuffed Animals

(Marie)

Some experts on Alzheimer's say that activities for people with dementia should be adult in nature, but anyone who reads the stories I'm about to tell would have to agree there can be exceptions.

Adorable

Having seen Ed's pleasure at the 'Lee-tle' Yellow One during one of my visits, I asked, "Would you like a bunny rabbit, too?"

"Oh, I would love a bunny rabbit!" The next day I took him a bunny rabbit, which he immediately named Adorable.

I had to go out into the hall to talk to one of the nurses. Before leaving, I put Adorable on the foot of Ed's bed. When I came back, I saw that he had put Adorable on his pillow. I was touched.

Ed looked me right in the eyes again and said, "Maybe I'm 'see-ly' at my age playing with these 'Lee-tle' stuffed animals, but I r-r-really do love them so much."

Seeing how much joy the little animals brought him, I kept taking more and more, and he loved each one more than the one before.

The Breathing Puppy

I was in the mall a couple of weeks later and saw a battery-operated puppy. Its little chest moved up and down as though it were breathing. I was sure Ed would love it, so I bought one for him. In fact, it was so cute I almost got one for myself, too!

Ed loved it as much as he loved all the other stuffed animals.

One day he told me, "The first thing I do when I come to my r-r-room is look to see if the 'Lee-tle' puppy is still breathing."

Again, I was deeply touched and so pleased that I had made him happy.

Art with Mary
(Daniel)

Here are some recollections of art therapy sessions that took place as part of the University of Alabama Honors Seminar, Art to Life, developed by Cognitive Dynamics Foundation, which I founded and directed.

The course pairs students and persons with Alzheimer's disease. They have an enriched relational experience, using art therapy and reminiscence to reveal and preserve the people's life stories and promote empathy among the students for individuals experiencing cognitive impairment.

In our second art therapy session, six students, a graduate journalism student, and our student facilitator for the course were in attendance. An art therapist conducted the session.

One time, our participant was Mary, a ninety-five-year-old with Alzheimer's disease, nearly sightless from macular degeneration, but with one of the most joyful and enlivened spirits imaginable.

Before the session, the therapist had talked with me about the challenges of artistically engaging someone with poor eyesight. The therapist had decided to try shaving cream art with Mary because of its use of the tactile sense.

Mary was always warm, and she reached out to everyone in the room. In each session, she started out by telling us how grateful she was to be there, to be included, and about how she was afraid she talked too much during the sessions. She also confessed she couldn't see well. As we delved into the session, she said many times, "Oh, this is just fabulous!"

The therapist started the session with some discussion of Mary's life, which flowed very naturally. Mary told us details about her family, and we reviewed some of the life story she had told us at the previous session. She told us about her father's cotton farm and about how the cotton used to be used for airplane wings. She mentioned that her husband had been a pilot.

When the art activity started, Mary sat at one end of the table, and the students filled the rest of the space. (The tables were placed in a 'T' shape.)

The art therapist instructed Mary about how to squirt shaving cream into an aluminum pan, choose her food coloring, place drops of her favorite colors in the shaving cream, and swirl the colors around in patterns of her choosing with a small wooden stick. Then the therapist told her to blot a piece of watercolor paper into the mix, absorbing the color. At last, she was supposed to scrape off the shaving cream, leaving beautiful patterns of color in an abstract form.

Mary sat eagerly and affirmed her interest. (Everything about Mary was affirming.) She had some help from the students, as she said she really could not see any of the details or colors. She chose red, yellow, and green food coloring, and her students helped her place the colors. The therapist then placed the wooden stick in her hand, and Mary made the patterns. The paper was blotted and Mary, with help, scraped off the shaving cream.

What happened next was miraculous, and I will never forget it.

Ingeniously, and with much compassion and empathy, the therapist suggested to Mary that since she was having trouble seeing the art, each student would be asked to comment about what the art meant to them and share those comments with Mary. After their comments, Mary would be in a better position to title her piece of art.

We went around the room and each of us told what the art made us think of, what we felt when we looked at it, etc. When the last person had shared his impressions, Mary was asked to title the art based on the students' comments. Quite obviously moved, Mary said she thought 'Celebration' would be a good name. Then, in tears, she said something I hope I never forget:

"There's something there…a new beginning."

She told how she had thought that she would never be able to create art again because of her poor vision, and that art had meant so much to her in the past. She began to speak of how wonderful her life had been and how grateful and full of joy she was about God's goodness in her life.

Although she could not see any of us, Mary told us how much it meant for her to know we were all feeling the same thing and that we were all experiencing the power of art to kindle relationships.

She said, "I want you all to know it, to really know it, every one of you, how important this is! I am so thankful."

During this experience, Mary told us that memories were flooding her consciousness, filling her with gratitude. She spoke tenderly of her wedding day and how the minister had started a custom that was apparently not in use at that time. Namely, having the bride and groom turn and face each other to exchange vows. As she talked about turning to face her husband and exchange the promises, she cried.

There are many other details that came out that day. It seemed that the storehouse of Mary's heart had been unlocked. The students were well attuned to what she was saying. All were completely present with each other and with themselves in the moment. Nothing else mattered at that time, and everyone was sharing memories of past events.

Mary said, "Lord, honey, I didn't know we were gonna have ourselves a prayer meeting today! The Lord sent you all to me. I know He did."

We all experienced the joy that is possible when visiting a person who has Alzheimer's disease.

I could say so much more about the importance of that day. Mary was validated in her current reality in that moment. She could create again, and she was so thankful for that. Her spirit and memory were awakened by the experience, and her life in that experience transcended Alzheimer's disease. Moreover, the experience kindled the life in each of us.

We came to bring something to her that day, but we also received the benefit, the honor, the blessing. What a great privilege to have had that experience!

After the event, one of the students said that in the car on the way home, she and her friends began to share their own vulnerability, to talk about their heartaches and trials, and to try and meet each other's needs. The student said that they were all perplexed at first, but then realized it seemed right to do this after the example set by Mary.

The students were entering into the vast expansive warmth of the self, which was shared in relationships with others. They were sharing in Mary's joy.

Thank you, Mary, for sharing your life with us!

The Beep Game (Marie)

I went to the Alois Center one day to visit Ed. I didn't really want to visit because my visits were boring at that time, and I was angry about Ed's condition. I wanted my old Ed back, but I knew that was impossible, so I had to force myself to visit that day.

Once I was there, I got an idea for a game to play with Ed. I started the visit by handing him one of his many stuffed animals, an act that always made him smile. I reviewed his growing collection and selected Adorable, the newest stuffed animal I had given him, for the purpose.

"Oh!" he said, his face shining as he stretched out his arms to take Adorable. "Oh! The 'Lee-tle' one! I love him so much."

He put Adorable to his face and kissed him. As always, it was as though it was the first time he'd seen Adorable.

Suddenly, I turned my head away from Ed and pressed Adorable's nose. I said, "Beep!" at the same instant.

Just as I'd hoped, Ed thought Adorable had said, "Beep." He looked at me, and his eyes widened as he marveled at the bunny's new ability. Then, he pressed the bunny's nose and I went "beep" again. He laughed, pressed the button repeatedly, and I said "beep" each time. I burst into laughter myself.

He laughed more and said, his voice full of wonder, "Listen what he does, Marie."

He pushed Adorable's nose and I said, "Beep."

"No, Ed," I said, laughing and deciding to reveal the secret. "I'm saying 'beep,' not Adorable."

"Oh!" he said. "You are wonderful. You are great. You are superb to make this 'beep' just when I press the bunny's nose."

He then exclaimed loudly and emphatically, "You could ask a 'hunnerd' people and they would all say you are magnificent."

He then repeated that sentence verbatim.

Next, he tried to trick me. He pushed the bunny's nose fast several times. I managed to keep up, saying "beep" each time. Then he suddenly slowed down, still trying to fool me.

He is really alert today, I thought.

After that, he picked up the 'Lee-tle' Yellow One, the first stuffed animal I had given him, and we played the same game with it. Ed kept praising me for being 'so magnificent.' We giggled like two young children playing together. It was fun.

One morning shortly after that, I realized I was actually looking forward to visiting Ed. I no longer felt bored, dejected, unloved, and unloving during my visits. I enjoyed them and left feeling emotionally satisfied.

Just seeing Ed smile and hearing him laugh had become more than enough to make up for losing some characteristics of our previous relationship.

Visiting Miss Daisy
(Marie)

"I've come to visit you, Miss Daisy," I said in a perky tone of voice.

"Me?" she exclaimed, smiling, looking up at me, raising her eyebrows and putting her hand over her heart.

"Yes, you," I answered, delighted by her excited reaction.

She already had won my heart. It was obvious she was thrilled to have me visit, even if she had no earthly idea who I was.

During that visit—our first—I discovered that Miss Daisy's social skills were so good you'd think she was volunteering to visit me!

One of the staff members had told me Miss Daisy loved Elvis, so I told her, "I understand you like Elvis."

"Elvis," she said with disdain. "Where'd they get that?"

"Well, what kind of music do you like?"

She blurted out, "Classical!"

"Who's your favorite composer?" I inquired.

I didn't really expect her to remember the name of any one composer, but she promptly and definitively said, "Tchaikovsky."

For the next visit, I wrapped up a CD of The Nutcracker Suite and gave it to her. She tore off the gift wrap, smiled broadly when she saw what was inside, and thanked me repeatedly.

After a few minutes, her eyes became downcast and she said, "I'm sorry I don't have anything to give you."

To help her save face, I pointed out, "Well, you have some cookies on your table."

She laughed lightly and said, "Sure. Help yourself."

When I soon asked if I could have another, she said, "Take as many as you want. They're from Hy-Vee. Hy-Vee has good cookies."

She was right! They were some of the best cookies I ever tasted.

Then, I put the disc into the slot of the portable CD player I'd brought along. It was immediately obvious that she was familiar with the selections. She smiled, moved in time to the music, and used her hand to tap out the rhythms on her lap.

She even knew when each piece was almost over, because she started clapping right before the last notes. Miss Daisy appeared to be more vigorous with each number. She loved every one more than the one before, and it was such a joy to see her exhilaration.

What's more, I loved it, too! I have a background in classical music, so we have that in common. It's almost as though we were destined to be paired.

At the end of the visit, she said, "I hope I see you again." Then she whispered, "But I probably won't be here. I'm going home tomorrow."

I knew full well she wasn't going home the next day, but had no intention of telling her that.

"Well, if you do go home," I said, "have a wonderful time there. But if you are still here, I'll visit you again next week."

"Oh, that would be wonderful," she said. After a couple of seconds, she repeated, "But I probably won't be here."

Then, as always, she insisted on walking with me to the front door. I moved beside her as she inched along ever so slowly, unsteadily pushing her walker down the short hallway. We said goodbye, and I left.

When I went the next week, she was in her room.

"I'm Marie," I explained, pretty sure she wouldn't remember me. "I'm a volunteer visitor here, and I've come to spend some time with you."

She studied my face carefully then said with a slight hesitation, "Uh, I think I've seen you before."

"Yes, you have!" I exclaimed. "I visited you last week."

"Oh. That's marvelous," she said.

Then we got down to business, to what would soon become our special routine. I ate cookies while we listened to The Nutcracker Suite.

In fact, all of our visits were the same. She gave me cookies, then we listened to the ballet suite. I did this because I knew she loved the music and wouldn't remember we listened to it the previous time. So I didn't have to think up different activities every week.

I so looked forward to my visits with Miss Daisy. And the smiles on her face said she enjoyed them, too.

A Puppy in a Pocket
(Daniel)

I probably shouldn't admit this, but I will, for any possible benefit you might receive from hearing it.

We had just navigated, again, one of those difficult transitions and had moved my father into a different specialty care assisted living facility (SCALF) unit. We had brought what things of his we could and arranged them in familiar locations in his room. We also had placed some identifying items of significance to Dad in the shadow box outside his room so that he could recognize the room as his.

This helped personalize the environment a bit and showed some of his life story to caregivers at the facility and those who visited him. It also helped remind him who he was when, on some days, it might have been hard for him to know.

I was struggling at that time, as well. We all were. Feeling inadequate and ill prepared to help my father and my mother with the challenges they were facing, I needed my own forms of therapy. I started writing and took up playing the piano by ear. I also decided it was time for our family to have some pet therapy.

I had at least one of every kind of pet growing up: hamsters, guinea pigs, white mice, rabbits, ducks, chickens, a pony, and cats and dogs, among others. My favorites were dogs. No matter what other pets we had around, we always had a dog. Dad loved dogs.

After I married and my wife and I moved away for graduate school, we got Mom and Dad a little beagle. This dog was theirs for a few years, but it met a tragic fate while chasing off a UPS truck. They wanted another dog but did not get one. I think Dad missed pets.

My wife, not having the affinity for pets that I did, required a bit of convincing. When I suggested guinea pigs for a start, Ellen said that we should just go ahead and get a puppy.

That we did, a little black and cream miniature dachshund we named "Heidi." Boy, is she cute! She was just a few weeks old when we moved Dad into the new facility.

I don't actually recall who had the idea (perhaps one of our daughters), but at some level, I confess I really wanted to do it. I wondered if pets were allowed in the assisted living unit. I didn't know, but one thing I was sure of: Dad loved dogs, and little Heidi just might be just the medicine needed to ease the pain of his latest transition.

At that time, Heidi could fit in the palm of my hand, so we devised a plan to take her in my pocket to see Dad. She seemed quite content in her tiny warm den, and I managed to make it down the hall and into Dad's room without anyone noticing Heidi.

We made our normal greetings, and Dad looked anxious and more confused than usual. When I pulled out our little Black and Cream, he changed instantly.

Most people with Alzheimer's can relate and respond to animals and children when they may not respond to anything else, and that is what happened. Dad reached for Heidi to pet her and talk to her and play with her.

He took the little dog in his big hands, and for a moment, I think his mind was free of the SCALF unit and back in the carefree days of his youth. It was a beautiful sight to see.

Dad's response to the dog also facilitated an interaction with his granddaughters and with the adults who were in the room. With the puppy as the centerpiece, we each entered into a playful interaction that was innate to all of us.

The dog had touched a deep place in my father and enabled us to tap into that same space.

When people are engaged at a spiritual level, meaningful relationships will result. This is not dependent on the cognitive state of the ones participating in the relationships. I think Heidi was able to connect to Dad's spirit.

A man and a dog. That's all it takes, really.

Remember the power of pets to reach deeply into the being of people who have Alzheimer's disease and other dementias. Bring them a pet. But not necessarily a puppy in your pocket!

Gifts Can Bring Joy to a Person Who Has Alzheimer's (Marie)

Everyone loves getting presents, and typically people living with Alzheimer's are no exception.

I first learned this from Ed, who—when I gave him a new pair of shoes one day—exclaimed, "These are the most beautiful shoes I've had in my entire life!"

My knowledge of the value of giving gifts to people with Alzheimer's has been reinforced by experiences with some of 'My Ladies.'

One day, I took Ethel a small wrapped gift, just a decorative note pad with a magnet on the back and a pen attached with a string. I thought she would like it because she was always writing down things to help her remember them.

When she saw the present, her whole face lit up.

She was so excited that I was afraid she was going to be disappointed. As she was beginning to unwrap the gift, I told her, "It's just a small gift, Ethel. It's no big deal."

Her response was touching.

"I know, Honey, but it's a present."

By that, I think she meant she was happy to get a present no matter what it was. I think she meant that getting presents is wonderful.

Another of 'My Ladies' is Ruth. Ruth loves big-band music, so I took her a CD of Glenn Miller. She was ecstatic when we listened to it, and it was a true joy to see her so happy.

Still another of 'My Ladies' is Sue. Sue loves reading the newspaper, so I take one to her every time I go. Whenever she sees me, she gets a big smile on her face and reaches her arm out to take the paper. Sometimes I think she enjoys getting the paper as much, if not more than, seeing me.

Here's a tip. I always wrap the presents, even if they are little things you might not ordinarily wrap, such as a couple of cans of Dr. Pepper I took Ruth. She really enjoyed tearing off the wrapping paper.

You should be prepared, however, for a gift to be instantly set aside and subsequently ignored.

You see, some people living with Alzheimer's apparently enjoy seeing and unwrapping a present more than they actually enjoy having it. I think that's because they immediately forget about it once they've opened it.

That's what happened with another gift I took Ethel. I knew that religion was very important to her, so I took her a CD of hymns.

She enjoyed opening the package but then pushed the CD aside and spent the next five minutes asking me questions about my portable CD player!

"Where did you get it?" she asked. "How much did you pay for it? Do other people have one?"

She then repeated those same exact questions two more times— and in the same order. The CD player fascinated her and held her attention far longer than the CD did.

Since I had four 'Ladies' at that time, it began to get a little expensive, even if I did take just little things. So one by one I started 'stealing' back the presents I'd brought and giving them again at a later time. Thus far, I've gotten away with this. No one has ever remembered I previously gave them the same present.

As before, they just love getting and unwrapping the gifts. The gifts bring them joy for a short time, and that's what matters.

Skipping Rocks
(Daniel)

In July 2003, we realized that if we were ever going to take another trip as a family with my parents, we had better take it then. We wondered how much longer Dad would be able to travel.

Coastal Maine was one of those locales where we had always intended to go but never had gone. So we loaded up our two young daughters, my caregiver mother, and my father with early stage Alzheimer's and headed for the untamed, spray-shrouded coastal crags of New England.

We flew to Portland, rented a minivan for the week, and started up the coast, packed to the hilt.

The drive was breathtaking. Dad was an outdoorsman who felt most at home in the woods, and this is one reason we chose Maine. He tended to get a bit anxious and restless, and we thought the waves, winds, and the lilting of fir trees would be calming to his spirit.

We stopped frequently to explore, and as we traveled father north, it seemed every stop had a drop of a hundred feet to the crashing surf and rocks below.

As you would imagine, my mother and wife experienced a quite serious level of angst as our daughters and their Papa trekked out on the rocky cliffs for a view of the wild Atlantic waters.

I'm not sure who was keeping whom from slipping—three-year-old Maria, seven-year-old Julie, or seventy-five-year-old Papa.

As I watched each of my daughters take one of his hands and head toward the water, I remembered those days when I had done the same. When Dad and I had fished and waded and watched and yelled for an echo in reply by seas, lakes, rivers, creeks, and bays.

And we had engaged in what may have been one of Papa's favorite pastimes: skipping rocks.

My father had to have been one of the most skillful rock skippers who had ever stood on a shore. He could make one sail in a perfect trajectory, glancing the surface at just the correct angle to skip along with unbridled velocity, often reaching the farther shores of lakes or rivers.

He seemed to get tremendous satisfaction from it and never tired of it. This was part of what was innately him.

Daydreaming about this, I suddenly came to and looked up to a familiar sight. There was Papa, stooping down for a smooth rock to skip, showing the little girls how it was done. Problem was, the water was a little rough to be conducive to rock skipping.

Dad didn't care. He was having fun like he used to, searching for smooth stones with little friends to teach and help.

Truth be told, Dad was restless while we were driving. He was a little agitated when we were in restaurants or other public places. However, once he got out on the rocks with the little girls, he melded with the moment. He became serene, sinking into the deep clefts and crags of himself.

And the roughest waters that crashed couldn't touch him there.

Standing in the wind, playing with his granddaughters and looking over the surf, he drifted out in freedom from the moorings of an unrelenting Alzheimer's mind invasion.

He was sailing free in the ship of himself.

Even though this place was foreign to him and surrounded by danger, and he had just been confused and anxious, he showed his true self through an activity that was so much a part of him.

He was enabled, not disabled, standing there by the lighthouse and by those whom he loved.

After we arrived home and Dad returned to Caring Days, in his art activities he began painting scenes from Maine's coast: lighthouses, trees bending to the wind, sail boats, and sea gulls. The images and experiences had stayed with him.

I like to think the positive emotions attached to those times stayed with him, as well.

Why did he enjoy skipping rocks so? Was it the thrill of unending skips or the anticipation of reaching the farther shore? I don't think so.

I think it was the hands he held between the skips; the ones he helped to find the perfect rocks; the misty memories that just may have surfaced of another little child and another old man on another shoreline.

Skipping rocks had brought his boat back to dock in the familiar harbor of home.

The Alzheimer's Perspective on the Birds and the Bees (Marie)

Ruth is my favorite 'Lady.' As I have said, I realize I shouldn't have a favorite, but I do. Visiting her is special. She's incredibly good natured and often quite amusing.

It happens that I had published an article on the Alzheimer's Reading Room website about Molly Middleton Meyer, the founder of Mind's Eye Poetry. Molly is an expert at facilitating the creation of poetry by individuals and groups of people with Alzheimer's. She helps them use their memories and imagination to create stunning poems.

One day when I was visiting Ruth, I got the idea for us to write some poems together. From my interview with Molly, I'd learned that was something people with Alzheimer's could actively participate in and also something they enjoyed doing.

I had no special skill or experience in creating poetry with a person who has Alzheimer's, but I didn't let that stop me. Although I couldn't even begin to facilitate the creative process the way Molly does, I did hope I could work with Ruth to write some simple poems.

After visiting for a few moments, I asked her, "Do you like poems?"

She blurted out, "Oh, yes! Happy ones!"

So we decided to write happy poems. I didn't know exactly how to proceed, so I developed my own approach. I decided to simply start off by saying what I thought would be a first good line for a pleasant poem, then raise my right arm toward her and look at her expectantly as though to say, "You say the next line."

Although my procedure was very different and much simpler than Molly's, it worked extremely well. Ruth and I typically alternated lines—I'd say a line, then she followed with the next.

What surprised me was that in most cases she immediately spouted off a line that not only logically followed mine, but also rhymed with it. I soon realized that Ruth is actually better and faster at rhyming than I am.

As we went along, I wrote down our poems on a little sheet of paper. Our first one was about the birds and the bees. I thought that would be a good topic for a fun poem. Here it is:

<u>The Birds and Bees</u>

The birds and the bees

Crawl on their knees and

Do as they please.

They don't have fleas—

Those birds and bees.

The very minute we finished, a buzzer went off. An aide stepped in and told us there was a tornado drill and that we had to come immediately to the center hall. We had to sit in the hall for a long time, and Ruth got quite annoyed. I was kind of bothered myself.

So when the drill was over and we went back to Ruth's room, we decided to write a poem about the drill. Lines two and four were Ruth's.

The Drill

The drill

Was no thrill.

Give me a pill

And forget the drill.

That pill of a drill.

We created another poem during my next visit. It was based on the fact that Ruth loves my little Shih Tzu puppy, Christina, whom I frequently take on my visits. Ruth doesn't remember my name, she doesn't remember that I visit every week, but she remembers I have a puppy.

This poem is more serious than the others and is one of the few that doesn't rhyme. Ruth came up with lines 2, 4, and 6.

Christina

I love Marie's puppy, Christina.

She's friendly and makes me smile.

When she comes to visit

She checks out the room.

And I'm happiest

When she rests in my lap.

Seeing how happy Ruth was to participate in writing the poems, I decided we'd keep doing it. One day I'm going to type them all up and put them in a colorful binder for her. I'll make another one for myself to remind me of Ruth's joy while doing this simple activity.

Puppy's Magical Visit to a Memory Care Facility (Marie)

I've always heard that pets often can reach people with Alzheimer's on a level people cannot, but I was not at all prepared for the profound reaction my little puppy brought about during a recent visit to Ruth, a grand dog lover.

When I arrived with my itsy bitsy Shih Tzu puppy, Christina, Ruth said, "Oh, my sakes. Isn't she adorable! She's so tiny. Look at that cute little face!"

Ruth laughed when she saw Christina and had the biggest smile on her face I'd seen in the year I'd been going to visit her.

Christina, ten weeks old and weighing in at just three pounds, hadn't yet had her first haircut and was a little ball of fuzz. Her eyes peeked out from beneath a broad tuft of fur; her tail never stopped wagging.

The minute Christina saw Ruth, she jumped up on Ruth's legs, eagerly begging to be petted.

Ruth leaned down and petted Christina energetically.

"What's her name?" she asked, laughing again.

"Christina," I said.

"Christina. Oh, my sakes! What a wonderful name for this darling little puppy."

"You can hold her if you want."

"Oh, really?" she asked. "Do you mean you'd actually let me hold her?"

"Sure. Call her over to you and pick her up."

"Okay. What's her name?"

"Christina," I patiently said again.

Ruth sat down and called out, "Christina, come here."

Christina jumped up and romped over to Ruth, who immediately scooped her up and put her on her lap. Ruth's eyes twinkled; she was absolutely radiant.

She playfully ruffled Christina's fur and patted her solidly on her back. As though passing out a reward, Christina planted several wet puppy kisses on Ruth's face. The last one landed squarely on her mouth.

I was mortified and yelled—more loudly than I'd intended—"Christina, stop it!"

But Ruth just laughed and said, "Aww. She isn't hurting anything."

Then she said, "Thanks for the picture of her you gave me last time."

She pointed to the wallet-size photo of Christina sitting on her bureau right next to the picture of Annie, Ruth's Labrador who now lives with Ruth's son.

The strange thing is that Ruth had forgotten I'd brought Christina on a previous visit. The other odd thing is that I had no memory of having given her the photo. I guess between the two of us we managed to remember most things!

"Thank you so much for bringing her. I love her!"

Then we played a game with Christina. Ruth sat in the well-worn easy chair at one end of her room, and I stood at the other end just in front of the door.

Ruth clapped her hands and called, "Christina." Christina went racing toward her then dive-bombed her feet like Babe Ruth sliding into home plate head first.

The second Christina arrived, Ruth flung both arms straight up in the air and shouted, "Whee!"

Then I called Christina, and she shot back to me like a mighty steer in a stampede.

We both laughed so hard we were doubled over.

We called Christina back and forth like that for a good five minutes. Each time Christina dive-bombed Ruth's feet, and Ruth threw her arms up and shouted "Whee!"

Ruth and I never would have tired of it, but poor little Christina was worn out and laid down right between us. Then she put her chin on the carpet and looked up at Ruth as though to say, "I love you!"

I was pretty sure Christina wanted to be petted again, but she was too tuckered out to jump up and beseech us.

"Thank you so much for bringing her," Ruth said for the second time.

Christina was out of breath and her little pink tongue was hanging out, so I asked, "Ruth, could I get her some water?"

"Of course," she answered, and I went to her sink to get the water in a plastic cup.

After drinking copiously, Christina was ready to frolic again, so we resumed the game.

Given Ruth's shaky memory, I thought I could probably bring Christina frequently, and every time would be like the first time. What a wonderful gift that would be. So much pleasure for Ruth and so easy for me to do.

Finally and reluctantly, I told Ruth, "I'm sorry, but I have to leave now."

"Oh," she said, thrusting out her lower lip and looking downward. "Can't you stay a little longer?"

"I wish I could," I said wistfully and honestly. "I don't want to leave, but I'll come back to visit you next Thursday."

I was as disappointed as Ruth that I had to go. I easily could have stayed there another hour, sending Christina back and forth incessantly, but I had three 'Ladies' on my list to visit, and I needed to go on to the other two.

As Ruth walked me to her door, I was thinking that after such a vigorous workout, Christina was going to sleep well that night. I kind of thought Ruth would sleep well, too. And so would I.

Ruth and I hugged, as always.

"Thank you so much for bringing her," Ruth said. "What's her name?"

"Christina," I said again.

Then she proclaimed, "This is my best day since I've lived here!"

Lessons Learned from Visits with Special Activities

1. Music and the other activities we have discussed may reach people with Alzheimer's on a deep level.

2. People with Alzheimer's may remember and be able to sing all the words to familiar songs, even when they don't talk anymore.

3. Music, art, and other enjoyable activities may leave those with dementia in a good mood after the activity has ended, even if they don't remember the activity.

4. People with Alzheimer's may enjoy child-like toys and playing child-like games.

5. People with Alzheimer's may enjoy activities they didn't like before they developed the illness.

6. Even the simplest activities may bring joy.

7. Keep your sense of humor when interacting with a person with Alzheimer's. The joy of shared laughter forms a beautiful bond.

8. Some people with Alzheimer's retain excellent social skills.

9. Simple gifts may bring joy to a person with Alzheimer's.

10. Wrapping the gifts may increase their joy.

11. People with Alzheimer's may enjoy listening to or helping write poems.

Chapter 15: Stories About Moments of Lucidity

<u>My Gift</u>

> For you, this gift I give:
> to know the inward being
> and be known.
>
> Daniel

Those Stunning Moments of Total Lucidity

Introduction

Many people who have cared for someone with Alzheimer's can tell you amazing stories about their loved one's moments of lucidity. These precious events can last for anywhere from a few moments to several hours or even most of a day.

Marie has a friend whose mother actually had an entire week of clarity. Her mind was clear as a bell for seven days, then suddenly she returned to her former state of dementia.

No one knows why these episodes happen. As a person's illness progresses, however, moments of lucidity tend to occur less often, so when they do happen, it's all the more striking and precious.

We know from personal experience and the experiences of other caregivers that those moments of lucidity are usually joyful and provide an opening for meaningful relationships to occur.

We feel that the gift of our complete attention and presence and the lending all of our listening skills to the interaction may help to create an environment where lucid times are more likely to occur.

The following stories are a few surprising examples of lucidity we have witnessed.

An Intuitive Knowing
(Daniel)

A couple of years ago, I had the pleasure of visiting with Naomi Feil, who developed Validation Therapy, for an on-camera discussion that explored the personhood of individuals with Alzheimer's and other dementias for an upcoming documentary. I learned so much from her vast experience with this population and thoroughly enjoyed her stories.

One story she told was about a very old woman who came to a group activity looking happier than usual.

"Mrs. Jones, you have a big smile today. Tell us why!"

"Oh, I'm so happy. I just had the most wonderful conversation with my mother and my aunt. I simply didn't have the heart to tell them that they were dead."

Feil speaks of the levels of knowing we all have and the deep awareness that remains even in those with dementia.

"As people age and experience cognitive impairment, they may lose some of their logical and chronological thinking," Feil explains. "But the deep knowing is still present."

Mrs. Jones knew at some level that her mother and her aunt had passed away, but experiencing relationships with loved ones who have been vital elements of one's life can fill needs that may be difficult to express.

Feil says that family members of elderly people with cognitive impairment who hear illogical statements like the one above may assume that personhood has been lost, but this is not the case at all.

Needs have to be expressed and dealt with. Mrs. Jones needed to 'see' those loved ones again and perhaps needed to feel known and loved and accepted.

The way we respond to statements like the one from Mrs. Jones will play largely into whether we are able to experience joyful visits with persons who have Alzheimer's, or whether we leave such occasions feeling sad, frustrated, or even grieving over lost relationships.

First of all, we should attune more to the emotional content of what a person with dementia is saying than the factual content, which may be erroneous. Building an interaction upon the energy of the person will be much more fulfilling than attempting to reason with him about facts.

Mrs. Jones led us to her happy place. Why would we want to lead her in a different direction?

Second, we should emphasize the good and de-emphasize the bad.

In Mrs. Jones' scenario, the warmth of good conversation with loved ones is pitted against the fact that those loved ones are no longer physically present. When visiting those with dementia, we should put energy into exploring the relationship through reminiscence, then bringing those positive memories into the present, not commiserating over the 'bygones.'

Again, Mrs. Jones took us by the hand and led us into the joys of relationships. Let's not dig in our heels!

I have no idea what it must be like to live with the confusion and unfamiliarity of dementia, though I realize that I may someday find out. However, I can imagine that it would be soothing to retreat into the safe embraces of dearest loved ones and friends, even if I know at some level that they have long-since departed.

To be with them again might just be the right 'dose of medicine' for my 'dis-ease.' I would probably know more deeply what it is that I need than anyone else, and I don't believe that will change if I have dementia.

The fact is that if we want to be able to have joyful visits with people who have Alzheimer's, we have to believe they are still persons who possess a 'knowing,' a deep inner intuition or awareness that may not at first meet the eye.

This 'knowing' may have very little to do with their orientation, short-term memory, or language ability—cognitive functions that are commonly lost due to Alzheimer's and other dementias.

If we believe this intuition remains, then we can follow them where they are taking us, and we may just gain some insight and understanding ourselves that we didn't have before.

After all, they are the ones who are navigating through this maze of confusion and found enough light to illuminate the smiles on their very own faces.

"You'll Get the Job!"

(Marie)

I had applied for a grant writing position at the American Academy of Family Physicians. I'd just had a successful phone interview, and they were inviting me for an in-person one.

I assumed Ed wouldn't understand what I was saying when I told him about it. A few weeks earlier I had mentioned that I was looking for a new job, and he reacted with utter incomprehension. I could have told him that day that I did my laundry or went to the dentist or fell down the stairs. It would have been all the same to him.

When I arrived to visit that day, I went directly to Ed's room. When I entered, I found he was in his bathroom so I sat down in the rocking chair to wait for him. I was suddenly overwhelmed with sadness. Here I was with the best news of my entire career, and I couldn't share it with the person I loved the most.

Soon he came out, a determined look on his face, steadily pushing his walker, feet moving in deliberate, evenly measured steps slapping down on the linoleum floor. Janelle had dressed him nicely in the beautiful navy cardigan I had given him one year for his birthday, navy Dockers, and a pale yellow shirt.

He greeted me enthusiastically, told me how happy he was to see me and how beautiful I was. He maneuvered to the sofa and moved aside two big bunnies so he'd have a place to sit. Then he picked up 'the Lee-tle' Yellow One, ever his favorite stuffed animal, put it on his lap, looked at it affectionately, and started 'padding' it.

"I have to tell you something that's very important, Ed," I said, mindlessly picking up Adorable, another of his animals.

"Oh, please. Tell me!" he said, continuing to 'pad' the little animal.

"Well, the American Academy of Family Physicians has a job opening for a grant writer, and I applied. It would be a wonderful job for me," I said, rocking back and forth and keeping my words simple.

I stopped rocking and waited for his response, expecting something totally unrelated such as, "It's nice that we live here in Romania," or "Your shoes are so beautiful," or "That lady on the television is the Pope."

But he didn't say anything like that.

"Oh! Marie! They will hire you," he said, putting the 'Lee-tle' Yellow One down and looking me straight in the eye. "With your background and qualifications," he went on, "with all your experience and the tremendous success you've had over the years, they will certainly hire you!"

I just stared at him, dumbfounded.

"Don't worry. You will get the job," he continued immediately, his eyes tearing up. "I'm so happy for you, Marie," he said, his voice cracking a little. "I'm sure they'll hire you!"

I was profoundly touched. Not only was he talking like the highly educated man he was, he also cared about me so much that he had tears in his eyes just thinking that something good was going to happen to me.

"Congratulations!" he said. "You will get the job. I'm one hundred percent certain!"

"Thank you," I whispered. "It's my dream job."

I didn't know what else to say. For that brief moment, I'd had my 'old Ed' back. What a precious and unexpected gift.

Dogs Are Very Selective

(Marie)

A strikingly handsome young man was signing out as I entered the Alois Center with my Shih Tzu, Peter, one day. The man's general demeanor led me to believe he was a successful professional. He had jet-black hair, dark brown eyes, and a strong jaw.

"What kind of dog is that?" he asked, smiling at Peter more than at me.

"He's a Shih Tzu," I answered. "His name is Peter."

"I'm Tom Brooker," he said, extending his hand.

"Oh. You must be here to visit your mother."

"Yes, I am. I was just leaving. And you know what? My mother loves dogs. Would you do me a favor? Could you take Peter to see her? She's in the Terrace. Her name is Denise. She doesn't talk, walk, or feed herself anymore, and rarely makes any sense on the few occasions when she does say a couple of words, but I'm sure she'd love to see Peter."

"Sure," I said. "I'll stop on my way to visit my friend, Ed."

I entered the Terrace, found Denise's room, and peeked in. A woman with short, straight grey hair was lying in bed and wearing a thin, off-white nightgown. Her eyes were half closed, but she seemed to be awake.

"Mrs. Brooker," I called out in a soft voice. "Are you awake?"

She opened her eyes fully and nodded 'yes.'

"Hi," I said. "I'm Marie, and I just saw your son in the lobby. He asked me to bring my dog to see you. This is Peter."

"Oh! Wonderful! I love dogs."

I was astounded that she'd actually talked.

Since she didn't sit up or anything, I picked Peter up and held him near her. Peter immediately licked her face. She laughed and petted Peter.

"Gee, I'm surprised," I said. "He doesn't usually kiss people he doesn't know."

"Dogs are very selective," she answered, her lucidity astounding me.

I had the feeling it was probably the most lucid statement she'd make for a long, long time. That was confirmed, in fact, by her son when I told him about it the next time I saw him.

Moments of Clarity
(Daniel)

Toward the end of my father's life I watched *The Notebook*, a movie based on the book by Nicholas Sparks, and I finally understood something.

I had seen Mother and many other caregivers striving to tease out moments of clarity, of recognition, of special memories that could be shared even late into the course of Alzheimer's. Something that would restore, if only briefly, the spark of a relationship that had been present in earlier times.

In Sparks' story, a caring husband reads to his wife from a notebook she had written about their love story before she lost her memory, with the hope of seeing that spark, that light of recognition, so that things could be the way they were before.

It finally came, and I understood.

After Dad had transitioned into a residential care facility, Mother continued to visit him lovingly and diligently. During those visits, she would try to remind him of who he was through reminiscence, as well as by speaking with him about family, friends, important milestones of their life together, happy occasions, etc.

She would speak to him about their wedding anniversary, about who his best friends were, about joyous family get-togethers and trips, and similar things. During the last few months he was with us, Dad became less able to respond with words and often just blankly stared at us. In fact, verbal responses became rare during those late visits with him.

One day while Mother was at the facility, she was reminding Dad of their anniversary, of his birthday, and of his best friend's name. Dad was offering no response.

Finally, she asked, "Lester, honey, how old are you?"

Briefly, the fog cleared and Dad's spirit and sense of humor lit the room.

"Not as old as you!" he replied, saying nothing else for the remainder of the visit.

We have laughed and laughed about that over the years, and his response taught me a lot.

One thing it showed me was that people with Alzheimer's may be much more aware than we think they are, even late in the course of the disease. We should never say anything in their presence that could be upsetting, make them feel 'less than normal,' or have any effect other than to be of comfort and build them up in their present state.

It also showed me that essential traits of personhood still remain. Dad's sense of humor was always keen and endearing, and there it was, still making us laugh.

He was also a man who possessed a good bit of pride for who he was and in his appearance. He still carried a comb in his back pocket well into the course of Alzheimer's, and kept that full head of white hair looking sharp. In reality, he was six years older than Mother, but that day he may have felt the need to assert his youth again.

Most importantly, I have learned that memory and recognition are not essential for meaningful relationships and joyful interactions. Relational energies are found at a much deeper place.

It is not necessary to develop a connection based on remembering facts, faces, and events. However, it is essential to get in touch with the humanity of another by tapping into our own humanity.

We must make ourselves vulnerable, open and uncluttered, willing to enter the present moment with no judgments or expectations, except that of finding another person who needs us.

It is true. They may not appear to remember us, and this will hurt. They may not be able to recall that special occasion that meant so much to us, but there they are, present with us, capable of a deep connection. In fact, they need one.

Gently touching, singing a favorite song, maintaining eye contact and smiling, holding a hand, and having compassion and shared affection in the moment can prove that joyful interaction is still possible.

And thus come our own moments of clarity.

Wearing It for Death

(Marie)

My mother had died just three days before I made this visit to Ed. As I walked toward his room, I realized I wasn't looking forward to seeing him, because I didn't think he'd understand when I told him my mother died.

I certainly didn't expect him to be able to comfort me, as he would have even a year before. I prepared myself for his absence of empathy.

I found Ed sitting in the rocking chair dozing, so I called his name. It surprised him and his head bobbed up. Then an instant later he recognized me, and a smile came to his face.

"Oh! Marie! It's you. I'm so happy to see you. You are so beautiful!"

After a few minutes of small talk, I decided to tell him about my mother. I was certain he wouldn't remember her, even though they'd met several times over the years and had liked each other. Like me, she'd been especially attracted to his charming accent and his distinct European manners.

"Ed," I began, feeling sad just thinking about Mother. "My mother died last week. You remember her? You met her a few times."

He looked up from his favorite stuffed animal, Adorable, whom he was 'padding.'

"Honestly," he said after a few seconds, "I don't remember her, but I'm very sorry she died."

I gave him a prayer card bearing her photo. He turned it over, saw the praying hands on the back and thanked me several times for showing it to him. I also gave him the eulogy I had written. He studied it for a long time. Since his ability to read was very limited, I wasn't sure how much of it he could understand, if anything at all.

"This is very beautiful, Marie," he whispered. "You should be proud of yourself for writing such a lovely eulogy."

Then he read the last sentence out loud perfectly.

"In closing, Flora often said, 'I've had a good life, and when I'm gone I don't want you kids to cry.' To that we kids say, 'Sorry, Mom, we tried to honor your request, but just can't do it.'"

"Just can't do it," Ed repeated, the paper quivering in his ever-shaky hand. He looked up at me and said it once more, "Just can't do it."

Then he put the prayer card and eulogy on his nightstand.

When I left, I said, "I'll come back again tomorrow."

"Oh, I am very happy to hear that," he said. "Wonderful! Marvelous!"

I had been a little worried that perhaps telling him about Mother's death might make him think about his own death, but I realized he probably didn't have the capacity to make such links any more.

"Ed, you remember I told you my mother died?" I mentioned the next day.

"My mother didn't die," he said, looking baffled. "I just talked to her last night."

I knew, of course, that his mother had been dead for decades, but I wasn't about to tell him that.

"No, Ed," I said. "I'm talking about my mother. My mother died, not yours."

"My mother is fine," he said, still confused.

I dropped it.

Three days later, casually dressed in black jeans and a black cotton turtleneck, I was sitting with Ed as he ate his lunch of unappetizing-looking pureed something or other and tapioca pudding. I was so distraught over Mother's death, I'd decided to wear a black blouse or shirt every day for a month.

When he finished eating, he put down his spoon, looked directly in my eyes, and said, "You look so beautiful in that black shirt, even though I know you're wearing it for death."

I was simply stunned.

You're Always in My Heart

(Marie)

One time my dear friend, Rosa, was going to come to the Alois Center to visit Ed with me. It was a cold November day, and I arrived first. I rushed into the building to escape the bitter wind that was blowing leaves in wild circles around the parking lot; they looked like tiny leaf tornados.

I looked for Ed. When I didn't see him, I figured he was in his room.

I was an hour early because I wanted to make sure Ed was awake, shaved, and dressed. I pressed 4421 on the keypad and entered the Terrace hallway. The first person I saw was the aide, Janelle. I was delighted she was on duty that morning. She was my favorite aide.

"Hi, Janelle," I said as the door automatically shut behind me. "Ed's going to have a special visitor this morning."

"Oh! Wonderful! He loves company. I'll get him all fixed up like a gentleman. He is a gentleman, you know? That's what he is, alright. A gentleman. He should look like one, too."

We stepped into Ed's room.

"A good friend of mine is coming to visit you today, Ed."

"Oh, I'm delighted," he said. "Is she your mother?"

"No, she's a good friend. Her name is Rosa."

"Oh. Rosa," he said. "That's a lovely name. Is she your mother?"

"No, Ed," I calmly answered again. It was clear he didn't remember he'd just asked me that. "Rosa is my friend."

As if on cue, Rosa burst into the room. Wearing casual black slacks and a brilliant magenta blouse that matched her vibrant energy, her presence filled the room with an air of excitement. She had dark hair, even darker eyes, and constantly gestured with her hands as she talked, making it easy to guess she was part Italian.

Emotional by nature—and culture—the visit was special for her. She wanted to connect with my Ed at the deepest level possible, given whatever his mental status might be that day.

After I introduced them, Rosa sat on the sofa beside Ed. They took off, having a lively discussion, Rosa gesturing and Ed motioning with his shaking hands. It was as though they were lifelong friends who hadn't seen each other for a long time. I was amazed. Ed was pretty lucid, except for his confusion about whether Rosa was my mother.

I realized it was going to be one of those precious times when, for some mysterious reason, he regained his faculties, if only briefly.

Ignoring me completely, as though I were an inanimate extension of my chair, Ed and Rosa suddenly stopped talking, held hands, and looked at one another. They didn't utter a word. They just held hands and gazed into each other's eyes.

Ed finally spoke. With the honesty and freedom of a child, he simply said what he was feeling.

"I'm looking at your face…I like it. You are so beautiful."

"I'm honored to visit you," she told him.

"Huh! I'm twenty times honored to see you."

I wondered how a man with dementia could make such a lucid, spontaneous, and emotional response to a total stranger.

Next, Rosa fished her wallet out of her enormous purse and showed Ed pictures of her grandchildren. Then she related a recent talk she'd had with her granddaughter, Jennifer.

"I told Jennifer," she said, pointing to Jennifer in the photo, "that when you love someone they are always in your heart and you are always in their heart, even if something happens to one of you."

She turned to Ed and said slowly and loudly, emphasizing each word.

"You're always in Marie's heart, and she's always in yours."

"Ma-r-r-rie's always in my heart…but I'm not sure I'm always in hers," he said.

"Yes, Ed. You're always in my heart," I assured him, patting him on the shoulder.

"Oh. I'm very happy to hear that."

Feelings were simple for Ed those days. His mind didn't delve into the complexity of others' emotions. He didn't have mixed feelings. He didn't have lingering doubts or suspicion about other people's motives. I told him he was always in my heart, and that settled it for him.

We talked for another five minutes, then Rosa left after numerous goodbyes, thanks ("from the bottom of my heart"), and hand kisses from Ed. I lingered. Ed said Rosa was a marvelous lady and asked if she was my mother. I told him she was a friend. Then I told him I had to leave, as well.

"When are you coming back?"

"Tomorrow."

"Wonderful! Marvelous!"

Lessons Learned From Moments of Lucidity

1. People with Alzheimer's may have moments of total lucidity.

2. We need to treasure these moments, however brief they may be.

3. People with Alzheimer's seem to have a deep level of intuition or 'knowing,' which we should honor in our relationships with them.

4. We can create an environment conducive to moments of lucidity by listening and being present.

5. We should recognize these lucid moments as open doors to the inner world of people with Alzheimer's.

6. Being willing to enter those open doors will increase the likelihood of building joyful relationships.

7. Though moments of lucidity are treasured, they are not necessary for meaningful relationships to occur. All that is necessary is non-judgmental presence in the moment, vulnerability, and need.

Follow Me

Follow me.
I know where the music is.
Come with me and sing.

If I miss a word, which I'm apt to do, don't worry.
The melody sings itself. You'll hear it, too.

What matters are the wordless harmonies we'll make
and whether we can find a way
to move together, tightly held.

They sent a warning starting out
that I will stumble—
ever falling forward into nothing.

But they didn't tell me
(because they couldn't know)
there would be a song for singing, dancing
with anyone who's not afraid
to hold my hand and meet me in the now.

Nothing won't be nothing
if we are one and bravely go there.
Love and joy will give that place a name.

    Daniel

Acknowledgments
Marie

I want to thank our editors, Carol Bradley Bursack, BA; Ellen W. Potts, MBA; and Mary Theobald, MBA, for their outstanding assistance and valuable contributions to this book. In addition, I thank the *Huffington Post* and the *Alzheimer's Reading Room*, both of which previously published some of the material in this book. And I thank Maria Shriver for allowing me to blog on her website as an "Architect of Change." I also would like to thank Brookdale Senior Living for the opportunity to visit My 'Ladies' at their Overland Park, Kansas, Clare Bridge memory care facility. My visits have enriched my life tremendously and added valuable material to the book. Finally, I wish to thank Dr. Potts for a wonderful collaborative experience.

Daniel

I am grateful for the life, story, and art of my father, Lester E. Potts, Jr., who courageously asserted his personhood when many would have thought he'd been rendered incapable of that due to his Alzheimer's. Likewise, I thank the staff and clients at Caring Days (The Mal and Charlotte Moore Center) who looked past the infirmity to see Dad's spirit, and for Dad's art teacher, George, who patiently shared his gift with my father. I thank our editors Carol Bradley Bursack, BA; my wife, Ellen W. Potts, MBA; and Mary Theobald, MBA, for their invaluable contributions. I also am grateful to the team at MariaShriver.com for publishing my monthly blog about Alzheimer's caregiving. Furthermore, I thank Dr. Marley for her invitation to collaborate on this project. Lastly,

I am grateful for the opportunity to be in joyful relationships with people who have Alzheimer's, through programs sponsored by my foundation, Cognitive Dynamics.

About the Authors

Marie Marley, PhD

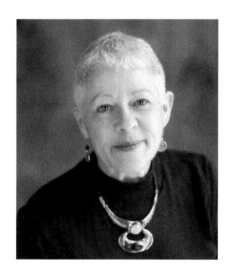

Marie Marley was an expert grant writer who, over the years, acquired a keen understanding of many geriatric topics, including dementia. However, none of that could have prepared her for the sometimes difficult demands of loving and caring for a person with Alzheimer's disease.

The touching story of her lifelong relationship with Edward Theodoru is narrated in her uplifting, award-winning book, *Come Back Early Today: A Memoir of Love, Alzheimer's and Joy*. The book focuses on the time when Ed had Alzheimer's.

Marie blogs regularly on the *Huffington Post*, the Alzheimer's Reading Room, Maria Shriver's Architects of Change website, and other Alzheimer's websites. She has published more than 250 articles on Alzheimer's caregiving on these sites and has made presentations on topics of interest to caregivers at support groups and professional meetings.

She lives in Kansas City with her little Shih Tzu, Joey, and her new puppy, Christina. Ed would have been so delighted to meet them both.

Daniel C. Potts, MD, FAAN

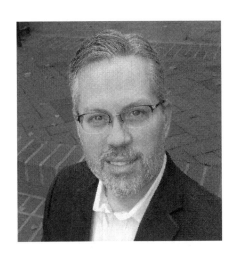

Daniel C. Potts is a small town boy from Aliceville, Alabama who became a neurologist and loves to write and tell stories, sing, take photographs, enjoy nature, and celebrate the wonder and beauty of life on earth.

His father's inspirational story of emergent artistic talent after the diagnosis of Alzheimer's disease set Daniel's life on a new course: to tell the story of the human spirit, which triumphs despite disease and disability, and to share hope with others.

Daniel has told his father's story through his dad's art and his own poetry in *The Broken Jar*, and has since published six books of poetry and photographs celebrating art, nature, and the human spirit. In addition, he was editor-in-chief of *Seasons of Caring: Meditations for Alzheimer's and Dementia Caregivers*, published by the Clergy Against Alzheimer's Network.

With his wife, Ellen W. Potts, MBA, Daniel wrote *A Pocket Guide for the Alzheimer's Caregiver*, which is recommended by Maria Shriver, the Alzheimer's Association, and the American Academy of Neurology. One of Maria Shriver's Architects of Change, Daniel blogs monthly on her website, MariaShriver.com.

Daniel's foundation, Cognitive Dynamics, makes art and other expressive therapies available to honor the life stories of persons with Alzheimer's and other dementias. For his work in Alzheimer's advocacy, the American Academy of Neurology (AAN) designated him the 2008 Donald M. Palatucci Advocate of the Year. Daniel is an AAN Fellow, the organization's most esteemed category of membership.

An affiliate faculty member at the University of Alabama College of Community Health Sciences, the University of South Alabama College of Medicine, and the UAB School of Medicine and a sought-after speaker, Daniel now practices neurology at the VA Medical Center in Tuscaloosa, Alabama. He resides with his wife, Ellen, daughters Julie and Maria, and miniature Dachshund, Heidi.

Appendix: Works Cited

Avadian, Brenda. Finding the Joy in Alzheimer's: Caregivers Share the Joyful Times. Pearlblossom, CA: North Star Books; 2006.

Bell, Virginia and Troxel, David. The Best Friends Approach to Alzheimer's Care. Baltimore, MD: Health Professions Press. 6th Revised Printing; 2006.

Brackey, Jolene. Creating Moments of Joy for the Person With Alzheimer's or Dementia: A Journal for Caregivers. Lafayette, IN: Purdue University Press. 4th Edition; 2007.

Brenner, Tom and Brenner, Karen. You Say Goodbye and We Say Hello: The Montessori Method for Positive Dementia Care. Create Space; 2013.

Clergy Against Alzheimer's Network. Seasons of Caring: Meditations for Alzheimer's and Dementia Caregivers. Create Space; 2014.

Feil, Naomi. http://www.vfvalidation.org. Accessed August 30, 2014.

Larkin, Carole. "10 Tips for Communicating With an Alzheimer's Patient;" Alzheimer's Reading Room. http://www.alzheimersreadingroom.com/2010/03/ten-tips-for-communicating-with.html. Accessed August 10, 2014.

Marley, Marie. Come Back Early Today: A Memoir of Love, Alzheimer's and Joy. Olathe, KS. Joseph Peterson Books; 2011.

Marley, Marie. Marie Marley's Web site. http://www.ComeBackEarlyToday.com. July 2011. Accessed January 1, 2015.

Meyer, Molly Middleton. http://www.MindsEyePoetry.com. Accessed September 14, 2014.

Potts, Daniel C. and Potts, Ellen Woodward. A Pocket Guide for the Alzheimer's Caregiver. Create Space; 2011.

Snow, Teepa, Senior Gems Table. http://www.seniorhelpers.com/pdf/Senior_Gems_Tips.pdf. Senior Helpers Website. Accessed January 1, 2015.

"A New Page in O'Connors' Love Story." USA Today. November 12, 2007.

Made in the USA
Lexington, KY
19 May 2017